Notes on the Journey:

Living with Sarcoma & Hope

Laura A. Koppenhoefer

ISBN: 978-0-692-29886-2

Editors -- Lyle Ernst and Ann Boaden

Cover designer -- Ken Small, www.digitalbookdesigns.com

Cover photo -- Courtesy of Sheryl Davis Svoboda

Photos in book -- property of Laura A. Koppenhoefer

Printed in the United States of America

Published by Living in Hope Publishing

Printed by Total Printing Systems, Newton, Illinois

DEDICATION

To Erica and Sarah:

God bless you.

I love you.

CONTENTS

FOREWORD

By Mohammed Milhem, MD

"The art of medicine is to amuse the patient and let nature cure the disease"...... Voltaire

Sarcoma makes up 1% of all the cancers in the world, approximately 10,000 patients are afflicted with this disease every year in the United States. Being a sarcoma physician is a rare entity in itself, given that there are 150 subtypes of the disease, one truly needs a wise mind to navigate such difficult and rare cancers. An important trait is one of collaboration which is paramount to the success of treating such a difficult disease. Given how rare sarcoma is, each individual that is plagued with this disease is a hero that uniquely battles the lack of knowledge created by the hard reality that we do not understand this disease. Laura's efforts put forth in this book offer a unique view of such a fight.

For those of you who have ever watched a Dr.Who episode on TV may understand how I view sarcoma patients; perhaps more as companions traveling through space and time while experiencing the rare opportunity to be part of something far greater than we can possibly understand while considering the greater question about the mystery of life and the reasons why things happen without reason or explanation. That is the feeling that sarcoma gives me: a difficult disease that does not touch many but those it does reach are transported into a different world.

Laura is an amazing woman and one with a strong attitude and faith that has helped her fight against cancer since receiving her diagnosis in October 2011. In her story she shares much more than the cancer fight that many of us are used to reading, while offering a unique look at a rare and uncommon cancer diagnosis handled with dignity and grace.

Laura attests the lack of knowledge of a disease by those treating her cancer through thorough discussion and a greater understanding while working as a team that can come together locally, regionally and nationally through collaboration to better treat patients.

Laura delivers a very inspiring story as you walk with her through her experiences as a patient dealing with a very rare sarcoma diagnosis. She demonstrates a deeper patient-related perspective of her 3 years as a patient with a disease yet to be understood.

Mo

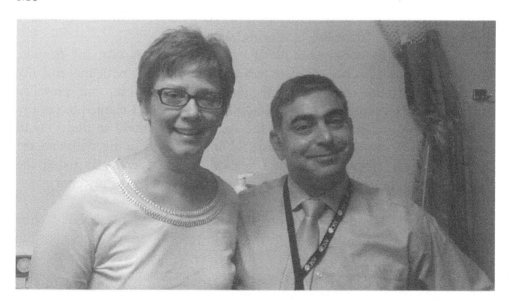

We're all smiles because we are fighting sarcoma. Laura Koppenhoefer and Dr. "Mo" Mohammed Milhem in the Holden Cancer Center at the University of Iowa Hospitals and Clinics in Iowa City, Iowa.

INTRODUCTION

Welcome to a conversation which started in 2011 with me and a "box for my story" on the web site called "Carepage.com." It is still a conversation with me, but it is also a web-based conversation with 850 family, friends, and friends of friends. It is sometimes a conversation with God -- usually in prayer, usually with questions, and more often with thanks. It is not a conversation with cancer -- in my case stage four sclerosing epitheloid fibrosarcoma -- but it is because of that cancer that I write.

In this Carepage conversation, I would write something called an Update every so often. People would read that and could write responses. I was used to people reading and hearing what I wrote because I was a pastor. However, these were different kinds of conversations. It wasn't about someone else anymore; it was about me.

I was pretty convinced that if I didn't tell my family, my friends, and my congregation about what was really going on with me and my cancer they would come up with their own plausible, but possibly inaccurate, ideas for what I was experiencing. Perhaps I wanted to get my own information, called "Notes on the Journey," out there so that I could "control" what people knew. I wasn't dying -- I was living with cancer! But most of all, I wrote because I needed their prayers. By using the Carepage, I could reach many people very quickly and save my energy for the long road ahead.

So why would I leap from the internet world to a book? For several years people told me how much reading my "Notes on the Journey" helped them. Maybe they had cancer too, or loved someone who did. Maybe they were going through some other life challenges. Maybe they wanted gardening tips or someone to commiserate with on the depth of the snow, parenting young adults, or disability paperwork. (All included here...) Maybe they just wanted to walk along with someone else who was striving to connect their faith with daily life. Regardless, I kept saying "No" to their idea to publish these pages.

Then, during one visit with my oncologist, he spent a lot of time talking about the need for sarcoma research. You'll read about that here, too. This book is in your hands as my contribution toward ending sarcoma. My initial goal is $20,000 -- that is enough money to fund two clinical research trials at the University of Iowa in Iowa City, where I receive my care. I want *us all* to make a difference in the direction of these little known, rare cancers called sarcomas.

I hope this book is a support to people who are living with sarcoma. I live with sarcoma *and* hope. You'll learn a lot more about hope in this collection of Updates from the Carepage entitled "LauraKoppy Notes on the Journey." Again, welcome to the conversation.

PROLOGUE

My name is Laura. I am a Child of God. I am the mother of two wonderful daughters, Erica and Sarah. I am an Evangelical Lutheran Church in America (ELCA) Pastor. I am a friend to many.

Yesterday, September 28, 2011, I learned that I am also someone who is living with cancer.

I am awaiting confirmation of the exact type of cancer, but it appears to be a type of sarcoma. As I am learning, this is a very rare cancer, but it takes about 150 forms. On Friday, September 30 I will have a surgical biopsy to determine the exact type. On October 11, a Tuesday, I'll meet with my oncology team to learn what my treatment will be. Know that I, like you, am much more than my cancer. Know this as well...God walks with us all.

Living with Cancer

From November of 2010 I have had pain that went down my right leg with extreme exercise. In January of 2011 I started "doctoring" for this pain. It seemed to be a part of some back issues....some arthritis, a small bulge in a disc (L4-L5). I did many months of physical therapy, epidural injections, and water physical therapy. Nothing helped. My loving, observant mom noticed as I was moving my youngest daughter to college that my right hip seemed swollen. I pointed out that swelling and my increasing sciatic symptoms to my local orthopedist and he ordered an MRI of my hips (a broader MRI than what I had when my back was scanned). A large mass in the right gluteal muscle of my hip showed up. My orthopedist referred me to University of Iowa Hospitals & Clinics in Iowa City and I went yesterday with my mom and dad. While I went in confident that no cancer would be found, I was wrong. Dr. Buckwalter, the orthopedic surgeon, and then Dr. Milhem, the oncologist and their amazing staff, tested and scanned and told us what is happening.

The mass in my hip is most likely a sarcoma. This cancer has also spread to my lungs. Something, maybe just fibroids, is going on with my uterus.

Dr. Buckwalter is very confident that he can remove the mass in my hip. (This would be GREAT, as it hurts, my leg hurts, it is hard to sleep/walk/sit/play competitive games/enjoy my recliner for lengths of time/do the hokey-pokey with my usual grace/garden/trim the hedge (which isn't all bad)/carry groceries/shop for long periods of time, etc...you get the idea).

Here's the trick: the most important place to get at is the lungs. I have NO idea what the treatment plan will be. October 11 is the day to find that out. Nobody says "this is how long you have to live." Please don't ask. I don't know. However, I find that I do a fine job of living 24 hours every day, and plan to keep that up. I expect you all to do the same. Dr. Mohammed Milhem (Dr. Mo as he is called) is wonderful. He is a sarcoma specialist, one of about 70 in the United States. If there is a treatment to be known or used or anything, he knows it. Period. I am 100% confident in him, his team, and in Dr. Buckwalter. I suggest that you be confident too.

I appreciate prayers....especially for my daughters, my parents, my brother, and my mother-in-law and my whole extended family. Pray for the congregation I serve, Trinity Lutheran Church in Moline, IL -- they are wonderful people of God. Pray as well for my friends....too many to list I know they are very concerned.

And this happened. When I was in the Oncologist's office, or rather just walking into the office, I started crying. I couldn't believe I was there. I would rather have been anywhere else. When I got to the registration desk, I couldn't speak to say my name. I just stood there and cried. The woman at the desk was wonderful. She used humor (which I respond well to). She gave me chocolate (that helped). Then Mom, Dad and I waited. They had a puzzle table area, so Mom and I worked on that puzzle, sort of like the puzzle we are trying to put together to get me well.

As we sat there, a woman came over and said she saw me crying when I came in, and asked if she and her prayer group could pray for me, and what was my name... I said "Yes, please yes, my name is Laura." I asked her her name and if I could do the same. Her name is Ronnie...and yes she would like that. So, I ask that you pray for Ronnie as well. Please.

The exam room we went to next would start me down a familiar path of grief. In 2004, my husband of 19 years, Rodney died after a 6 month battle with colon cancer.

What do I know now? I'm not alone. God is here and through prayer, so are all of you.

And, on October 5, 2011, I turn 50. I am celebrating. Birthdays are good. Fifty never looked so good.

2011 UPDATES

Overwhelmed
Posted Sep 28, 2011 7:28 p.m.

I am overwhelmed....
~by the prayer, support and care of my congregation, my family and friends...and their congregations too.
~by the ministry of my congregation in offering a prayer vigil for me tomorrow Thursday and Friday. I am humbled and proud and thankful .....
~by offers to help in so very many ways
~by yellow....it turns out that this is the "color" for sarcoma (not the cells in the body but the color for popular support like pink is for breast cancer).

(This was my favorite color as a little girl through high school and college. Yellow was also Rod's favorite golf shirt color and flower color. I feel his presence, love and support through this all. The yellow mums are blooming in the back yard and so is one yellow rose on a bush that hasn't bloomed for weeks. And, now as I look, Erica's toenails are painted yellow too. Isn't it amazing how something so simple as a color can convey help and hope?)

I am overwhelmed....
~by the effort of getting back with all of you....so I'm not going to be able to do that. I'm glad that I've set up a CarePage. I'm feeling a sensory-emotional-physical overload today. I guess I should have expected that.
~by the love and care of the staff at church. Please pray for Pastor Larry and for all of them. They give their all in what they do, and are picking up right where I may need to leave off for a day or a week or what ever. Pastor is stepping in for a wedding this weekend. This week is when the final installation of the pews, pulpit, carpeting and such is happening in our sanctuary. I am sad not to be able to be there. However, I am so very proud of our congregation for making these upgrades, repairs, hospitality efforts and esthetically beautiful changes to our sanctuary.

1

~by your love for my family, especially my daughters. I know you are praying for them.
~by God's continued presence. And, I am thankful.

Thankful
Posted Sep 29, 2011 3:08 p.m.

I am thankful....
~ that 5 a.m. only comes around once a day...that seems to be the toughest time...pain meds have worn off, not able to sleep, and non-helpful thoughts seem to rule.
~ thankful for the many prayers and smiles and everything that you all are lifting up for me and my family
~ thankful for Skype...so I can see Sarah in her dorm room at college
~ thankful that the ultrasound of my uterus is done this morning. From my non-expert opinion it looks like they are seeing some small fibroids there that have been there for some time.
~ thankful that times have changed from when I was a little girl when people did not even "say" the word cancer. My dear Grandma Harding used the letter "C" when she was talking about it. However, now, not only do we talk about it, smart people *do* something about it. I am thankful for the people who have been in studies and for their families who have walked with them so that I can tell my family (on October 11) what can be done for me.
~ thankful that God called and calls me to preach the Good News. Last weekend I lifted up the story of the resurrection....Easter morning...earthquake, tomb empty, guards "stupefied," Mary and the other Mary mourning and fearing, when a joyful, big bright angel tells the women to tell the men to get on to Galilee. Then Jesus shows up to them, too --woohoo! I imagined Jesus as the River of Life.... Have you ever seen a dam break or a levy open up? No one can hold back the water! The water can do nothing other than rush out! I see Jesus like that from the tomb--he would do NOTHING other that rush out to fill every space, go everywhere, and wash us all clean. That image of Jesus coming to me, to us, and to you is with me. Jesus is in this "whole thing" I am

2

experiencing, and may explain why I had to take a 50-minute shower yesterday. I guess that when I tell others the Good News, I tell myself, too.

~ thankful for the body and blood of Christ that Pastor Larry gave me in the Chapel this afternoon. I cannot think of a better meal. It is even better than lasagna! And that is saying something!

~ thankful that I *know* that this could be an even longer list.

(e.g., daughters, Play Doh, Fisher Price Camels, the yellow "Just Do It" Nike shirt that I am wearing to the hospital tomorrow)

Surgery time
Posted Sep 29, 2011 3:46 p.m.

Now, I have a time. God has already provided the people to be with me: *smart* doctors, great family, great pastor-friend, and also my dear brother Eric who is flying in from Mississippi to be with me tomorrow.

Surgery -- this is an "open biopsy" under general anesthetic. They will be taking out samples of the tumor so that they can figure out just what it is. Dr. Mo says we need to "give it a name" (by that, the name of the type of cancer). I have not named my tumor, don't feel a need to, and would probably just use that name to yell at it anyway.

When? 1:30 p.m. is the scheduled time. (I arrive there at 11:30 a.m.)

Where? University of Iowa Hospital

This is out-patient surgery...meaning I will come home after the surgery. Praise the Lord that they will let me have 8 oz of apple juice tomorrow some time between midnight and 11:30 am...whew -- it is hard to go hungry!

I think we can do this together. *Be strong and of good courage, be neither afraid or dismayed, for the Lord your God is with you whereever you go.* Joshua 1:9

Waiting

Posted Sep 30, 2011 10:02 a.m.

....waiting on the Lord....*Yet those who wait for the LORD will gain new strength; They will mount up with wings like eagles, They will run and not get tired, They will walk and not become weary.* Isaiah 40:31

....waiting to drink apple juice for a bit as I get 8 oz of something before 11:30 this morning (of course, I am also smelling the yummy scrambled cheesy eggs and toast that Mom and Dad and Eric are eating...they need their strength! (and it is pretty funny to tease them about eating in front of me)

...waiting to talk to the orthopedic surgeon about what position I will be placed in on the surgical table...seeing as most positions eventually become painful. (This would be a helpful "praying point," that I not have terrible sciatic pain in recovery.)...and ready...ready to tell you that your prayers are helping...I did not have *any* time this morning at 5 a.m. when I felt alone or apart from God's presence. I even woke up to texts and prayers. You all are good....and good medicine.

...ready to get on with this...

Home with some good news

Posted Sep 30, 2011 9:58 p.m.

Ok...you all are some *powerful* prayers...and we have a loving God...I am pretty heavily medicated, so I'm having my brother (the doctor) type the update....Many thanks....Laura

Laura went through the procedure well. Dr Buckwalter came to the waiting area and discussed the results. He said that the tumor was fibrous in appearance. The frozen sections did NOT appear to be consistent with a malignant sarcoma as initially expected. The sections favored a more slow growing benign tumor. PRAISE GOD!!! We will need to wait for all the slides to come back to know a specific diagnosis which will take about 7-14 days. We are cautiously optimistic. That brings us to the lung findings. Since this is not likely an aggressive malignant sarcoma, other causes of the nodules in the lungs arise. Laura has had significant lung infections in the past and these findings may be a result of these illnesses. Again, we need to wait for a final diagnosis, but feel we are in a much more hopeful position than 24 hours ago. Another encouraging note was that Dr. Buckwalter felt that the tumor could be removed without much difficulty. Even a benign tumor can grow around vital structures, but in this case it has not. The only significant vital structure in this area is the sciatic nerve and the tumor does not involve this nerve (it presses on it, because of its size, but is not growing into it). Thank you again for the thousands of prayers that have been offered up on behalf of Laura. We have all felt His amazing power and peace. .....Eric

Things that help
Posted Oct 1, 2011 12:32 p.m.

many things help....
~ my family here, including mom who got up with me 3 or 4 times at night to help me to the bathroom!
~ the prayers of so so many!
~ the yellow ribbons tied on my door, the swing, the frog watering can, the front porch posts, and more, to greet me as I returned home last night, and in the beautiful sunshine this morning.
~ hearing from the doctor that it may not be cancer...(this could actually be #1 through about a zillion)
~ getting to be optimistic (this is a preferred position of mine anyway)
~ good pain meds
~ the surprise lawn help this morning
~ the note from the prayer vigil folks with scripture and hymn references....all read this morning with great thankfulness.
~ seeing the list of your names. You make me smile and even shed a tear...(big surprise...right?)
thanks be to God....

Something to think about
Posted Oct 2, 2011 11:27 a.m.

So, it is Sunday morning. I love Sunday mornings. With the body of Christ at Trinity Lutheran I have especially been looking forward to *this* Sunday morning as we return to the sanctuary. Although I am pretty "thickly" medicated for the post-operative pain, I am still smiling, thinking about the sanctuary and the beauty of God and God's people in that beautiful place. I am right there in spirit.

I am reading through Philippians; this morning I am reading Chapter 4.

> *4 Rejoice in the Lord always; again I will say, Rejoice.*
> *5 Let your gentleness be known to everyone. The Lord is near. 6 Do not worry about anything, but in everything by prayer and supplication with thanksgiving let your requests be made known to God. 7 And the peace of God, which surpasses all understanding, will guard your hearts and your minds in Christ Jesus. 8 Finally, beloved, whatever is true, whatever is honorable, whatever is just, whatever is pure, whatever is pleasing, whatever is commendable, if there is any excellence and if there is anything worthy of praise, think about these things. 9 Keep on doing the things that you have learned and received and heard and seen in me, and the God of peace will be with you.*

I'm going to be reading and meditating on this in these next days. It seems like a long time to wait until Tuesday, October 11 to find out what is going on in my hip and lungs. Thinking only of that isn't going to help this time pass too quickly. It helps me to think of God's "nearness," and "peace that passes all understanding" and things that are "honorable" and "just" and "true" and "things worthy of praise."

Yesterday Mom harvested the patch of gourds, about 24 of them. They are just fun to look at. What a hoot! They are in a basket on my dining room table. They remind me that I planted them, months ago, and I am enjoying the harvest. In verse 9, what Paul reminds me of is doing the stuff I know how to do -- keep on doing those things -- to pray, to read scripture, to give and receive love in my family and friends, to laugh, to care for my body gently (even though I may want to walk around outside I need to avoid steps for a while!) Those are the things that will keep me on an even keel as I wait through these days.

Mom said that she thought I was doing a bit better last evening because I got a little testy about brownie crumbs on the kitchen floor. (This is probably true!) I also do think that this is a pretty "extreme" experience to go through to make turning 50 look good, but it has worked -- I think 50 is wonderful.

Wherever I go
Posted Oct 3, 2011 10:23 p.m.

My confirmation memory verse is a favorite....Joshua 1:9 "...*God is with you wherever you go.*" Physically, I'm not going very far very fast! I'm limiting myself to the first floor plus one step on the back deck. I tried to "back off" on the pain med this morning; however that didn't play out too well and I switched back up to two pills.

I find myself asking my family to tell me again and again how the doctor said that the tumor did *not* look like an aggressive malignant cell type. While this is exactly what I want to hear, it seems that my emotions are on a roller coaster, and have been trying to "out-run" God every so often. Tonight I feel a little achy and warm....not a level of temperature that sends me back to the doctor (I checked, twice) but one that reminds me to take it easy.

Your encouragements and stories and cards seem to be just what the doctor ordered. While I love Jesus, sometimes I need "Jesus with skin on," and so many of you are Christ in the flesh for me and I am thankful.

My family is getting a work-out with projects around the house, and with feeding me every two hours or so.

I think that tomorrow I will begin my reading with Matthew again...and the "no-worrying." I am reminded of a card that my Grandma and Grandpa Harding sent me many years ago when Rod and I were awaiting the birth of Erica in Portland. It read: *"We're not so very far apart. God can see us both."*

I do know this...with the help of God...and all of you...this whole burden is much lighter.

Joyful in hope at 50 years
Posted Oct 5, 2011 10:31 p.m.

Hope. That is what I chose for today. In the 1990s I was working at memorizing scripture. That has been a blessing to me...and interesting to see what the same scripture (God's living word) would mean to me over the decades. Today, it is Romans 12:12 *Be joyful in hope, patient in affliction, faithful in prayer.* Yep, that is where I am.

Today I could wrap myself in hope...mine and yours. It is easier, of course, to be hopeful when I get a good night's sleep, which I did last night. My eyes are filled with joyful images...flowers, my favorite salsa, a printed copy of the new springerle press that will be arriving soon in the mail from my daughters (which presses 16 cookies of carvings of the life of Christ), 50 frogs on sticks (put there by a team of seven, not four....three drove away as I came outside during their "escapade"), 50 "all dressed up camels," chocolate covered strawberries, a frog-fleece blanket, and prayers....countless, priceless prayers.

I will post a few pictures of frogs and camels....here are a few things to help "understand" them.

1) Frogs have significance for me, as I was called a "frog" by a bully in elementary school. However, years later as I was studying in Seminary, I received a simple gift from Sarah -- a pad of paper with "Fully Rely On God" complete with a cool frog picture on the cover. Then I realized that I am a frog...and that I do "F.R.O.G." as well!

2) The camel herd began with a wonderful gift of a Fisher Price Manger Scene a few years ago from my dear friend Penny. I have used it so much in my ministry. I pondered that maybe I am "part camel" as I take wise people to see Jesus on their journeys. The next year, she gave me a camel for each year I was old. (E-bay is almost as amazing as Penny.) The camel herd has been known to show up in confirmation classes, on sabbatical with me (Gamal, the camel, was pictured all over Israel and Germany), in

8

my office, in church programs (3-4 year olds are wowed by 49 camels, guaranteed.) She and my other friends also know my love of PlayDoh, and of marching bands (as a band mom). So, this year, my very creative friends dressed the whole herd in uniform (hats with plumes), gave them instruments, drum majors, and a flag team...and PlayDoh. It was just too cool. How could I be anything other than joyful?

It feels that with every time I get a card or text or what ever, that God keeps saying...I am here! I am here! I am here.....

On the mirror in my bathroom I keep this phrase...

"God made our location, his location. Good to be us." Amen

May I walk unafraid
Posted Oct 6, 2011 8:57 p.m.

This "day after the birthday" has been an inward journey.   Yet, I'm still focused on Hope. That is a good thing to do.

The other thing I tried to do today was to decrease some of the meds for pain. I had a very good night's sleep and I was ready. I did pretty well physically through the morning (except for nausea and dizziness) and with Cheerios I was better by lunch. This afternoon though, I've learned that there is a significant amount of cramping in my hip muscles and sciatic pain that had been covered by the meds. Maybe in a few days I'll try again. Part of my struggle in wanting to decrease the meds was my wild notion that maybe I could be fit to go back to church. (Never mind that I am not allowed to drive. I'm dizzy; I hurt. I don't fit in most of my clothes because of my hip swelling, and on, and on.) Some part of me equates "feeling a little better" with "getting right back in the saddle." I wrestled with this. Truly, I had learned better on sabbatical. I learned about rest and its healing power. However, I had underestimated the amount of emotional wrestling that comes with waiting to heal.

Fortunately three, yes three, dear pastors came to see me today. To hear my struggles. To affirm that my home is a good place for me to heal as I wait. To encourage me to be patient with myself. To reaffirm that I need to heal on the inside and out.

So, maybe this time of waiting is a retreat. A time to give and receive love. A time to trust in the Lord.

About two months ago I was on retreat with other dear friends on the Spiritual Formation Committee for our synod. I started thinking about this retreat today as I came across the words to a song from that day. After we sang we talked about what was on our hearts...what was it that we were striving to do. Today, my striving remains the same....to walk unafraid.

Let my prayers rise up
Posted Oct 7, 2011 9:21 p.m.

Today started with me pretty determined to find out what was going on with some gum/tongue/ear/throat pain. The nurse in Iowa City directed me to my local doctor, Anne Petre. Dr. Petre was great. Nothing was going on that will interfere in any way with what will happen in Iowa City next week (my great fear). I left with a flu shot, and thankfulness for Dad's chauffeuring and Mom to visit with during the waiting.

Home is still a place for praying. Affirming words and prayers are welcome. Those beautiful prayers rise up....like incense? That is not such a lovely image for me. I'm just too allergic. Anyway, today as I lay in bed trying to ward off a bit of medication "haze" I came up with a new idea for praying and aromas. What I smelled was a three hour stream of cupcakes baking. First chocolate, then vanilla, then carrot cake, then German chocolate. Erica was baking. Eight dozen cupcakes for my birthday party. She is a good good baker.

The ceiling fan in my bedroom, which is not far from the kitchen, kept the aroma in beautiful waves over me. Breathe in. Breathe out. Breathe in. Breathe out. When I breathe out, my prayers raise right up with my breath. Could it be that just as I breathe in those sweet scents and am reminded of its goodness, of my love for my daughters, that God breathes in our prayers? That our speaking to God in prayer....every flavor....is sweet to God? That God inhales our very breaths and says "Yep...I love this one...and this one...and this one...and this one..."?

This is an image I want to have today, because I am praying a lot. Not the quick "throwing it up there" kind of prayer, but the long, deep, pulled from my heart sort of prayer. The kind of prayer that is my "whole self" put in that prayer. The "Lord, I am serious about this" sort of prayer. I start to pray and it all spills out -- or up, actually. On this day it is a birthday cupcake sort of aroma rising up....breathed by God and then by me and then by God. Breathing and praying. Breathing and praying.

Showered with gifts
Posted Oct 8, 2011 10:46 p.m.

I am perhaps two exits beyond tired. I'm sure if I stay on this road there will be a toll to pay. However, hitting the pillow tonight without expressing thanks is more than I can do.

Today was the 50th birthday party for me that Erica has been planning since she graduated from college back in May. Seriously. However, if you saw what she accomplished you could see why it took so many months. Those cupcakes I wrote about yesterday--- soooo yummy, and very beautiful on a specially made 3-tiered cupcake stand. The food and decorations were wonderful as was the "shower" of gifts.

Guests donated $585 for Evangelical Lutheran Church in America (ELCA) World Hunger and $490 for Winnie's Place (our local homeless shelter for women and their children). Others donated directly to the ELCA Malaria Initiative in my name. I am honored by everyone's generosity. The "over ordered" fruit and veggies, a tray of each (plus about 2 dozen cupcakes) went to the shelter tonight. The shelter supervisor said they have women and many children right now, so the healthy food would help a lot.

I also want to congratulate those of you with stock in Kleenex and Puffs --- your stock has to have been driven up to the sky today. It seems that every time someone came in the door, I started to cry. How is it that the Spirit lives in (and drives all the way here from) places like the Quad Cities, Freeport, IL, Pontiac IL, Bloomington/Normal IL, Rochelle IL,

11

Champaign/Urbana IL, Rockford IL, Chicago IL, Morton IL, Seneca IL, Naperville IL, Wheaton IL, Hudson IL, Leroy IL, and Hastings, Nebraska!?!

Everybody kept telling me to sit down through the party, and mostly I did, but that is hard to do when my heart is just soaring. A friend of mine tells me that loving and being loved is like having the sun shining on both sides. She is right on.

During the party, a friend and brother in Christ, Bob Hansen, led a time of laying on of hands and of prayer...with an opportunity for me to offer my thanks for the gifts and love of those there and those there in spirit. I will never forget the warmth and weight of that touch on my head and shoulders. Again with the Kleenex/Puffs stock. I think that stock is up high enough. It is time to get well. I now have some new "Fully Rely on God" stickers and a Jesus action figure. I need to get back to work! I have cool stuff!

Action Figure Jesus and PlayDoh
Posted Oct 9, 2011 10:52 p.m.

I have always loved the Genesis 2 story of creation, where God walks in the garden, engages in conversation. This God kneels down and gathers up the dust of the ground and breathes life into it....and makes us. This is a very "hands-on" God. I, too, love getting my hands in the dirt. And I love the molding and making. Today, the new PlayDoh and the Action Figure Jesus (both birthday presents) got a work out with me and my elementary-aged great nieces, Taylor and Emma. When we got Jesus out of the careful packaging we found that his big moves were "positionable hands/arms" and "gliding action." We had no problem providing more moves and got busy building. We found Jesus in the churches we made. We found that Jesus said "Welcome" and "I love you" a lot. The more we talked about Jesus, the more hugs I got and kisses I got to give. Could it be that even just talking about Jesus helps us love one another better?

This sort of activity kept me from that wondering about what I will find out from the oncologist on Tuesday. I tell everyone who asks that my plan is to find out that this hip tumor is benign and boring, that my lungs bear the marks of my travels kind of like travel stickers on antique suitcases. Worn, but fine, just fine. I seek your prayers that my focus stays on loving God, being the healthy person that I am, and living the next 50 years with joy....and that the news on Tuesday will affirm that. I'll stop now so you can start praying...oh, who am I kidding? You are praying already...I can tell...

Carried by friends
Posted Oct 10, 2011 12:08 p.m.

One of my favorite stories of Jesus and the people who love him is from Mark Chapter 2. The word has gotten out about what Jesus is able to do...as well as hope about who he might be blows through the air, raising expectations for all of them. Four friends have a dear friend who is paralyzed. The four get their friend. No arguing. They just grab his mat with him on it and take him right through the town right to Jesus' house. Then of course, they can't get it in the house...too full. So they climb up to the roof, cut a *hole* in the roof and let their friend down through it so this friend whom they love can be right there...right in front of Jesus. And Jesus sees the faith of the *friends* and heals the man.
That mat is a precious place to be. I have carried many of you to Jesus. Now you are carrying me. I know Jesus can see your faith and hope and love. I can't think of a better place to be.
I have two appointments in Iowa City tomorrow to get the results from the biopsy surgery. There will be a lot of waiting. Of course, it will be fine, because you all have a hold of that mat.....and Jesus is right there.

13

Wherever I go today
Posted Oct 11, 2011 8:53 a.m.

I was ready to jump right in and say "Be strong and courageous, be neither afraid or dismayed, for the Lord your God is with you where ever you go." And then I remembered, "It is Erica's birthday! I need to make the labels for the house!" (We have a tradition of putting up little strips of paper with Happy #, Erica/Sarah.) So now I am back. There are "Happy #23 Erica!" labels all over the house with my mom's help. I have her presents wrapped and ready to open in the living room. But really there is only one present I want to give her -- two words, "boring and benign." That's all. I can't buy it. I can only receive it. Sarah's birthday is coming up in November. I want to give her the same thing.

I guess the gift I'll carry to Iowa City is God's grace. That's the gift we all have today. We can't buy it. We can only receive it. Grace sufficient for the day.

You all are doing a fantastic job of carrying that mat we're on. Mom & Dad, Eric and Erica are here with me. Let's go see Jesus for some healing.

Two names
Posted Oct 11, 2011 10:00 p.m.

The first is my name....Child of God. The second name is fibromyxosarcoma, the name of my cancer.

These are the highlights...(I am so tired and have explained this so many times, and have percocet-affected typing skills that this takes a lot of focus...)

1) This is a very slow growing cancer, also called a "low grade" cancer. High grade cancers grow super fast and have to come out right away. My cancer grows slowly and has been there a long time....at my guess four years.

2) Because it is a low grade cancer, it is not responsive to chemotherapy in the leg or the lungs. Chemotherapy works on cells that grow quickly.

3) The Plan: to remove the tumor in my right hip soon....likely late next week. The recovery from that surgery is at least four weeks.

14

4) The surgeon has some concern about removing 100% of the tumor because of its proximity to my pelvic bone (iliac crest) and sciatic nerve. Therefore he may not take 100% of it.

5) The Plan Part 2: to re-CT Scan my lungs at 4 weeks after my surgery to see if there is any growth. If none, we will keep watching and scanning. If it does start growing quickly, then there are some chemotherapy clinical trials that he could get me in.

6) Another possibility for the lungs is to do a resection (or surgical removal) of the small cancerous lesions.

7) Some statistics. Out of 100 cancers, one is a sarcoma. Out of 100 sarcomas, six are fibrous type sarcomas (mine is one of those types).

8) One more test is still not completed -- the cytogenetics (a type of genetic testing to see how this tumor "works" genetically....how it grows, divides). This should be in in a few days and may give more information.

9) How am I feeling? -- overwhelmed, but better after talking to the oncologist (Dr. Mo). At least now we have a name and a plan.

10) How to I feel about God? Just fine. I won't rule out being mad at some time or another, but I'm not mad now. I don't have a belief that God says, "You get cancer, and someone else gets this or that." We all get "something." I absolutely know that God was with us and stays with us. All the time. Period. This is Christ who went to the cross. I have no understanding of any god who sits on some throne far away, apart from my life or anyone's life. I still find that that mat you all held and continue to hold took me right to the people to whom God gave the gifts of healing. And, I am thankful.

11) What do I wish? That I didn't have to have the conversation with my daughters that I have cancer.

12) Is it real to me yet? Not really.

13) How do I feel about prayers? Keep them coming....it is good for you and it is good for me. God wants to keep the lines of communication open.

14) How am I healing from my first surgery? Very well with the incision....fair with the surgical pain, lousy with the sciatic pain. However my sense of humor is intact.

15) What the heck? 15? There is no 15....guess I just got carried away. If you read this far, bless your heart. Go hug somebody. Say your prayers. Get some sleep. I'll do the same.

Your best you, my best me

Posted Oct 12, 2011 11:07 p.m.

I have spent a lot of time lately around people who are completely being their best-selves. My mom and my dad come to mind. Honestly, I can't imagine my concern if this were happening to my daughters. And, my brother Eric. He is a tremendous doctor who's using his best knowledge, and compassion and care for me, his sister, who perhaps teased him mercilessly as "Ear-ache" when we were kids. He rocks. Just saying. Erica brought on her best party skills and currently is helping to organize my thank you notes as my "cloudy" med haze keeps those things from making sense. Sarah came home to bring me a joy that only she can tote around.

Each of you in your own way is helping. For some of you, it is that you check in, and hold me in prayer. Some leave a short note on the CarePage. Sometimes everyone can see those notes, sometimes they are just for me. You share my illness with your best praying people -- in your family, churches, friends. You name God's goodness and love. You tell me the way God is working in your life or tell jokes. Everyone is keeping cats out of my house. (Praise God.) Some of you are using words I actually said to you and yours in times of loss or stress. Those work for me and truly mean something to me, because, you see, I would only use my best stuff...the stuff I know, and mean, to you.

When Rod, my husband was diagnosed with stage-four colon cancer, and six months later died, it happened to him. I was as close to him as any person could be, but it was his body, not mine. Now it is my body and I'm sad.

Some day, probably soon, I'll be ready to pore over the internet to become the best former nurse former nursing educator current pastor expert on fibromyxosarcoma. But, not today. It took me a while in seminary to set aside my best nursing skills when I approached the suffering of a parishioner and to be the pastor in the room and not the health care provider.

Right now on this journey, I am the person and the theologian.

This particular cancer has so very very little information on it. Doctors don't say much about "how long." They really don't know.

16

However, people have known God for generation after generation. My best me has known God my whole life, so that is where I am starting.

What follows is my answer about the bright shining light of God and me, and the little light of my cancer (which is such a tiny little light....kind of like one bulb of a Christmas tree string at the 50-yard line of Rock Island High School's football field at noon on a clear day in July.) In other words, God's light is BIG....my cancer is teeny tiny in comparison)

These are things I hear some times....
1) "You are strong, so very strong, that you can handle this." Yep, I'm a pretty strong woman. I find that that whole praying to be strong and courageous (Joshua 1:9) after many months during Rod's illness made me realize that I was not strong as I needed to be going into something, but was stronger having come out on the other side. (I even went through a period where I stopped praying for strength because I wondered if it brought on more lousy stuff. I got over that.) I figure I may be strong now. I'll be stronger later, which brings me to....
2) "God never gives you more than you can handle." First, this is not Biblical. Second, the verse that people are most likely thinking of is 1 Cor 10:13, which says that God will not allow us to be tempted beyond what we can bear. Frankly I think I (we) am faced with more than I can handle *all* the time. The point is that the Jews of Jesus' time would never have imagined living a life where it is lived apart from God. All things are borne with God. All things. I think I (we) take on *much* more than we can handle *all* the time. This is my challenge....to make sure to use the help that is right in front of me all the time. (aka, Mom to change the water in all the flowers I have before she went home. For dad to take the broken light bulb out of the candelabra in the dining room. -- If you wanna see two people "light up"? Suggest that I do that on narcotics! Not!)
3) "Everything happens for a reason." I both believe and dis-believe this. I don't believe that "I got cancer" for a reason.....nope, not even to wax theologic to "readers." I am quite certain that God could have found another way to tell each of you that you are amazing and God loves you about one bazillion other ways. Probably you are each within driving distance of a church with a vibrant ministry that is making a difference in

17

your community where the "gifts" you have would make a positive difference in the lives of others.

However, I do believe that in every circumstance, God is saying "I love you" "I'm right here." I can think of messages or "ways" that God has spoken to me over the years. Sometimes God is quite subtle, like through the words of *just* the right hymn on a Sunday morning. Other times God seems to get right in my face and holler, like through *so* many people suggesting I should share my CarePages, combined with Dr. Mo's impassioned plea for sarcoma research funding. God is always talking to me and to you. There is a reason for everything....God wants us all to know we are loved and to love others as ourselves. I can look at leaves changing and just love them because they are pretty one day. The next day I look at the same tree and I see how yellow it actually is and in that pretty color be reminded how God is right there, right here, for me as well. That is a good reason.

4) "This isn't fair." Nope. Not fair. Rod had cancer. He died. I have cancer. I am living. Planning on continuing living until the day I die. And, I don't believe this "about" being fair. If this was all about fair, I would be done for. We all would be! I am a sinner, we are sinners, standing in the need of grace. Hope in the face of all of this, from everyday life to a crappy diagnosis, is what happened at the cross and the grave for me. Jesus rose. God wins. God is for me, for us. I will take Jesus' presence....Jesus' presence in my lowest, saddest, sitting in the chair two feet from the oncologist, over against any day without Jesus. I mean it. I think that today I will read Hebrews 11, the "Faith Hall of Fame." There are saints before us who have been through a lot too.

Things that help, Part 2
Posted Oct 13, 2011 7:07 p.m.

As I wait for the final call to tell me my surgery time I find myself frustrated. This doesn't help, so I've decided to focus on the stuff that does help. There's a lot of thankfulness. Here's some of it:

~ I do not have to have chemotherapy before having the tumor removed~ next week all (or most all, but please pray for *all*) of the tumor will come out.

~ I am closer to a time with less pain.

~ they will keep me in the hospital for at least one night to make sure the pain is controlled.

~ times of talking with others help.

~ prayer....yours and my own.

~ the palm crosses and the prayer shawls. The shawls keep me warm and loved on the drive to and from the doctor visits and surgery. The palm crosses have been in my purse and pocket....I remember reaching into my purse to touch the cross as the doctor was saying I had cancer...just to remind me that Jesus was there...and that God's love is bigger than any badness of any cancer.

~ seeing yellow in the trees, or pictures I've been given, or flowers or cards.

~ the risen Christ.

~ distraction

~ naps

~ comfortable underwear and pants (odd to list here, but boy it makes a difference in my pain level around my hip).

~ yummy food

~ my parents, my daughters, my family, my friends

~ the promise at the end of Matthew 28; *and lo, I am with you always to the close of the age.*

Mornings seem to be my most tearful times and this morning I needed to hear these words. In my old King James Version, the word "lo" is in this text. Lo is my nickname and I have always perceived Jesus speaking directly to me, but feel free to insert your name as well

~ the supportive staff and congregation at Trinity Lutheran in Moline where I am called.

~ the Acapella Sheep Quartet....a.k.a. four Fisher Price Nativity Sheep who have migrated from my church office, and are currently in Camel-flage --think camouflage -- on my piano....joy, joy, joy. (Yes, I do have creative friends.)

19

Wednesday at One

Posted Oct 14, 2011 11:53 a.m.

For over eight years, Wednesday at One has been the time of Bible Study and prayer at Trinity Lutheran. I started it and four senior pastors, one Children & Family Minister and I have led it using the texts for our preaching (or teaching) ten-days out ahead. I love that time, that study, and the people who have joined in on it through the years.

Now, that time, next Wednesday October 19 at 1 p.m. is my surgical time. In my scripture reading this morning I went to the beginning of the Gospel of Mark. Mark is the first writer of the Good News. I think about the immediacy of Mark for his audience. They were under persecution from without (e.g., the Romans, etc). I am under persecution from within (e.g., low grade fibromyxosarcoma). We both need to hear the Good News. We both need help with focus. We need to understand clearly what is asked of us as disciples. We need to understand clearly what this great gift of new life is and how to respond in love. Mark "cuts to the chase." I like that. Let's get on with the living, acknowledging that tough stuff is going on, but not overcome by that, not over come by that.....not over come by that.

One of my favorite scripture passages come to mind, 2 Cor. 4:16-18:
16 So we do not lose heart. Even though our outer nature is wasting away, our inner nature is being renewed day by day. 17 For this slight momentary affliction is preparing us for an eternal weight of glory beyond all measure, 18 because we look not at what can be seen but at what cannot be seen; for what can be seen is temporary, but what cannot be seen is eternal.

OBE, almost...

Posted Oct 15, 2011 10:26 a.m.

Pastor Larry Conway, a former military chaplain and my colleague in ministry at Trinity Lutheran, introduced me to "OBE" -- overcome by events. In ministry as in life, there are many OBE days. When I think hard about it, or if I go back to Dr. Buckwalter, the surgeon's exam room, or the operating room, I am a hair's breath from OBE. Yesterday I was "there" while I was here, in the recliner in the living room.

What helped? Remembering that there were some words, somewhere, in the writings of Paul that said I didn't have to be. What didn't help? I couldn't remember them. That is sort of the good thing/bad thing ratio of the meds I'm on.

Later I found those words and they were my companion the rest of the day, and this morning. 2 Cor. 4:7-12

7 But we have this treasure in clay jars, so that it may be made clear that this extraordinary power belongs to God and does not come from us.
8 We are afflicted in every way, but not crushed; perplexed, but not driven to despair; 9 persecuted, but not forsaken; struck down, but not destroyed; 10 always carrying in the body the death of Jesus, so that the life of Jesus may also be made visible in our bodies. 11 For while we live, we are always being given up to death for Jesus' sake, so that the life of Jesus may be made visible in our mortal flesh. 12 So death is at work in us, but life in you.

Last summer, I was at the Israel Museum in Jerusalem and got to see some of the Dead Sea Scrolls and parts of the clay jars that contained them all these thousands of years. We are even more fragile than those jars in the long term. They lasted a few thousand years already. We make it around to about 100. Both of us have the honor of holding the treasure...God's good news. Maybe I get it now. If God placed that Good News in only a few of us, that would be fool hardy. However, if it is placed in all of us, then it might just make it all those thousands of years...poured out, preached out, loved out, from jar to jar to me, who needs to be reminded again not to despair or become OBE.

Vertical
Posted Oct 15, 2011 2:57 p.m.

Saturday, later in the day....I'm thinking about denial. I'm wondering how much I am denying just to stay "vertical." I've also been thinking about friends who are in treatment...and friends who I know need to get something "checked out."

Do you know those platforms that are used to get our little kids a bit higher so we can see them in a program, or for speakers so they can be seen in a big room....or pulpits? I have one of those. My platform used to be my expertise as a nurse. Then it was expertise as a nursing educator. Then it was a pulpit. Then it was "Hey, my husband has/had colon cancer....get a colonoscopy everybody." I still have a pulpit, but now I also have fibromxyosarcoma. Now I don't think any family and friends would be very happy with me if I ran to my bedroom and did nothing about this. I am equally not happy about the people I care about who are not paying attention to their own bodies.

Sometimes I just remained frustrated because I try *so hard* to take care of myself. Most people know that about me. I do that for me, but I do it even more for my daughters, so they can see 1) how to do it for themselves and 2) so they know that I will stay with them, that I will not die early like their dad.

However, by caring so diligently for myself, I am physically in the best shape that I can be to heal. I have been kept from strenuous exercise because of pain, but I still have a BMI of 23.9. This is good. I am not stressing about "sweet snacking" now. I am eating healthy things (and actually crave them). And, I have an occasional Dove chocolate, or some of the yummy treats that people have brought to us.

These days I feel like I am making myself a beautiful spiritual faith-filled bed. I have had some glimpses of the pain that I have just under the surface. It looks much worse than my first scar. This bed is the one I will land in on the moments or days when I fall from this vertical stance. Thanks be to God....

Two directions...
Posted Oct 16, 2011 11:58 a.m.

I've thought of two directions I could go this morning...(Setting aside the direction of going to worship, which is where I *truly* wish I was, except for the fact that I cannot walk the distance to the garage and back without pain, and that the narcotics that I am on have me dizzier than a son of a gun, that I cannot risk getting the little cold/flu stuff that is running around....OK, yes, setting that aside.)
Direction one looks like this. Camels. The camel marching band that is so beautifully at attention on my piano in the living room takes offense at the words (intent) of Mark 1:6 where John the Baptist is described as dressed in camel's hair -- like that is a bad thing! As I have some of the most joyful and stylish and non-spitting camels that there are, I side with them and wish to correct the notion that being dressed in camel's hair is "ugly" or "uncomfortable" or "uncouth".
Direction two looks like this. I'm sorry. I am so incredibly sorry that I haven't quite figured out how to handle it. I have to include this second direction, because I know that there are so many that have dealt with more than their fair share of grief and loss and hurt and pain. I am sorry that the cancer that I have causes sorrow for so so many people. I know that it is "not my fault." But, I am still so sorry.
My sorrow took me to Lamentations, which I read *most* of, before wandering over and then back to 3:21-22 *But this I call to mind and therefore I have hope. The steadfast love of the Lord never ceases.* Do you know that crying on those thin pages of the Bible results in wavy pages?
In John 11:35 I find what folks think is the shortest verse in the Bible.... *Jesus wept.* (Confirmation students like to memorize this.) Really, in the Greek it means "Jesus began weeping" (Three words.) He wept because of the death of his friend Lazarus. He started weeping, not knowing how long he might cry. I get that.

Things that help, Part 3
Posted Oct 16, 2011 10:10 p.m.

The day passes and so do the tears. Things that help...
~ a delivery of a little cup of Cup 'o Joe Expresso ice cream from Whitey's (my Lord, this is a gift with definite healing powers. Note: This must be consumed in moderation as I have a milk allergy.)
~ prayers
~ talking with my mom with my brother on the phone
~ a hug of me, Erica and Sarah all at once this afternoon (Sarah had a weekend at home)
~ a walk (albeit a bit painful) to the zinnias in the yard and picking them for a bouquet and seeing the yellow at the center of every one of them....and the yellow of new leaves in bright contrast to the dried leaves that coat the yard
~ texting with friends and hearing the tales of my newest camel, Lolly on her trip to Valparaiso University
~ finding two sarcoma groups on Facebook, and a Listserve, to begin conversations with others on similar journeys....so far, no one with my exact cancer. One woman who posts because of the sarcoma (Ewings) of her son happened to have posted a picture of a golden yellow tree on Oct. 5, my birthday, on her Facebook site....
~ time in the kitchen arranging the beautiful flowers that have been in our home for many days.
~ remembering "God made our location, his location....good to be us...."

Roller coasters and Windows
Posted Oct 18, 2011 12:31 a.m.

A high school friend of mine, a seven-year survivor of a tough as heck non-Hodgkin's lymphoma, affirmed the roller coaster I am on.
Then he talked about windows -- windows of time. A window like today, or the time until my surgery, or the window of time until they rescan my lungs to see if there has been a change. He talked to me (and by that I mean emailed) about living fully in that window. What are the things I

want to accomplish? What does living fully look like? What are the memories I want to make with my kids, my family, my friends?

That got me off the recliner and off to arrange flowers and pick flowers and water plants. I was the only one home at the time. That work felt good for about twenty-five minutes, until I realized that I had overdone it, and was in some pretty stiff pain.

He didn't talk about balance, but I think that is a part of living in those windows of time.

I tried to think about what "window" scripture I knew but could only come up with 1 Cor 13 *"we see in a mirror, dimly , but then we will see face to face..."* Great. I know I can only get a part of the big picture now...and look forward to seeing my Lord...oh, what a day. But not today, or tomorrow! I am busy living this window of time and looking forward to the next one even if it has challenges in it.

Perhaps my next thought really is this.... *"Be content with* (I read *thankful* here) *such things as you have, for God, God's self has said I will never leave you or forsake you."* (Hebrews 13:5) Content/thankful for the joy I can find as I await surgery....spending time with friends, drinking tea from new cups, wearing great socks, pouring prayer over my daughters and folks, getting up off the recliner (when the dizziness stops) and looking out at the birds of the air and the black squirrels. There is joy in this window.

Surgery time change
Posted Oct 18, 2011 7:18 p.m.

Well, the roller coaster continues and the window is extended. My surgical time is now 2:45 p.m.

I have a bit of a concern with a scratchy throat, and am hoping that this is related to a little feasting that I did on chocolate yumminess (which is an allergy) rather than anything else.

Even though my time line is changed we have a God who is always there...(Psalm 121) so that *"the sun will not strike me by day or the moon by night"*......24/7/365.

Keep holding that mat...you are doing a good job....

Ready all carriers...

Posted Oct 19, 2011 8:00 a.m.

This is the day.

This is the day that Dr. Buckwalter takes out the tumor in my hip. I find myself repeating the last part of Matthew 28:20 *"Lo, I am with you always, to the close of the age."*

I'm up early this morning to have my one piece of dry toast and 4 ounces of juice. I did. Yum.

I'm in Luke this morning, the 5th chapter (17-26) and I'm reading his version of the healing of the paralytic. It is easier to get through the roof in Luke versus Mark's version, as there are only tiles. In this, I think Jesus sees all their faith...not just the carriers, but the carried as well. And, he calls the one on the mat, "friend." One of you reminded me that God's hand is on me and will be with me. A few years ago I had shoulder surgery for arthritis. I don't have pain in it and have full mobility; however, especially when it is rainy or the weather is changing, I feel a pressure on it, not too dissimilar from a hand resting there. I feel that today.

I am back on that mat today, or as Luke would say, my bed, a place to rest, carried by my friends and family. God can see your faith. God can see my faith. God is right here. God is our destination. God can heal and forgive. Thanks be to God. I'm ready to be healed. I'm ready to have people see me and be amazed at the healing. I'm ready to give God the glory and hope others will do the same.

Ready all carriers? As we say in our family, "You're doing a good job, and you look good doing it!"

Update...Surgery EARLIER!

Posted Oct 19, 2011 10:12 a.m.

I just got a call from U of Iowa Hospital....they want me there at NOON.

Being my best me
Posted Oct 20, 2011 3:48 p.m.

Hello, you great mat-carrying-praying-children of God....I am about 20 hours post operation. My best me has NO TUMOR in my hip! Woohoo! Instead I have a drain, and a pretty good sized owie, mmmmmany narcotics, and bad hair (really)....but a whole host of saints praying and an infinite supply of thankfulness. I am looking forward to feeling better, for sure. I have had physical therapy and walk (hobble with a walker) to and from the bathroom. I need to tell you that I *felt* your care on that mat yesterday and still today. I did not have anxiety...although my key people will tell you I got a bit testy when surgery ended up starting late. I even pointed a wrist ban scanner "gun" around willy-nilly as I waited for surgery.

Picking up my mat and walking
Posted Oct 20, 2011 8:43 p.m.

Hey there...this will be another short post....because
1) I am picking up my mat and WALKING, which brings on pain
2) of that pain....oh, my, goodness;
3) I will likely not go home until Saturday or Sunday.
So...the hip looks clear of cancer...final pathology will tell us that. The lungs....not clear.... but that scan at two months from the original scan is yet to come. Pain is lousy. Prayers are welcome.

A hair wash
Posted Oct 21, 2011 3:23 p.m.

That is the good news for the day....I got a hair wash (of course there is no dryer, but hey....)

I'm still pretty freaked out about the drain removal coming out at some time. Be strong and of good courage. Be strong and of good courage. Be strong and of good courage.....whew....
I can do this, and I ask God to help and guide me....

Another day
Posted Oct 22, 2011 11:12 a.m.

So....if I am sitting up, I can type a bit. My dressing was changed and I saw the incision...probably perfect for Halloween! My divot is right where I thought it would be....what a good sign that is....no 13 cm ball of cancer there!

Cheerios, Cheerios, everywhere are Cheerios
Posted Oct 23, 2011 7:13 a.m.

I am not kidding. They find my Cheerios pretty much everywhere....bed (of course), floor, over the bed table (so one aid threw it on the floor.....cracked me up), bathroom (whole container that was tipped onto the floor, not by me). Eating Cheerios....that is what I am up to at 5:48 am as I have had just had a BUNCH of meds and breakfast is an hour away at best.
One technician just came in to empty my drain. 40 cc since about 11 p.m. That is the big number to watch. It needs to be below 30 cc in some period of time (8 hours, 10 hours?) in order to have the drain out. I am still pretty nervous about this. I think I will try "casting all my cares on the One who cares for me."
And lest anyone think I would miss *any* opportunity for sharing the Good News, I do not. Usually I am telling the story of Jesus' birth because people wonder about the two camels standing on my over the bed table. This morning, my nurse was looking at the coloring page on the bulletin board at the foot of the bed. He said, "What ever is going on in that picture?" I said, "Well, it is a coloring page of an important Bible story for me." "Really? I'm not familiar with it." I told him it was the story of the paralytic, and then summarized it because he didn't know it. "Oh...that is

what that is in the picture...I thought it was some sort of puppet or marionette." Then I went on to say that a pastor friend had emailed me the coloring page for folks to do....it is therapeutic to color and all, and my mom colored that during my surgery. And, because she is a teacher, I gave her an "A+" on the page. Yep...I must feel better....preaching before 5:20 in the morning. Thanks be to God. Of course now I am four sheets to the wind........time to zzzzzzzzz.

Monday's random
Posted Oct 24, 2011 12:50 p.m.

Oh. My. Goodness, these medications have me in a fog! Regardless, they have me healing some more. I survived the hair wash I had yesterday. So....here's an attempt to organize my thoughts:
1) Erica has been here the last two days. Sarah has checked-in faithfully from college and wishes she was here.
2) My folks have been checking in on Great Grandpa Harding who is now in St. Francis in Peoria waiting for his INR to go down so he can have his lung(s) drained of some of the infection.
3) I really wish I could be with my grandpa....
4) (this truthfully would be about nine if I kept all the ideas that I typed while "micro-napping.")
5) My drain is still in.
6) The divot on my right hip is about the exact reflection (inward) of my other hip (outward).
7) This morning I was too warm in my room and had been wrestling with my covers. My nurse said that perhaps those "boots" that I velcro on to wear were pirate shackles....really? What a crack up! "Argh!" I said! "Avast!" I asked if any of my friends had paid him to use his best pirate skills this morning. Nope. The pirate joy was not lost on me, though.
8) Many a conversation has happened about the Jesus action figure with posable arms and gliding action which rests on my over the bed table as well.
9) Penny came by yesterday and brought Lolly the new camel. (or maybe it was the other way around) Regardless they were both there.

29

10) I also now have another IV location, no room mate (sad face here....I really miss my first one.

11) Next year = Cubs win. (What the heck...this is my list....)

12) I am always using my prayer shawls. They are loved! Hospital temps can be cool.

13) This being strong and of good courage takes some real focus and energy!

14) You really are a reader....good for you...you can go take a nap now......you just can't have mine...

Drain Out; Hurray!
Posted Oct 24, 2011 5:30 p.m.

Home tomorrow (probably, pretty certain, 99% sure) as I need to do "well" tonight.

Of course, as my drain came out, my 3rd IV site bit the dust....and I only have one more IV antibiotic dose to go.....honestly this is a pain in the neck as much as anything. I should have said this earlier, but a drain is a plastic tube with tiny holes in it, that is put in place during surgery, that is used to carry fluid away in the surgical site and into a "bagel-sized" case that I carried around the last five days.

So, the verdict on the "drain removal" is that YOU ALL ARE ROCK STAR PRAYERS! I mean, seriously, it did not hurt in ANY way. I feel well cared for, supported, and encouraged -- please know that I hold you in prayer as well.

Another leap of faith
Posted Oct 25, 2011 10:02 a.m.

Today, I get to go home!

I have a bunch of yellow post-its. They are the deep bright yellow ones, not the pale ones. They were sitting on my chest, the things I wanted to know about listed in tiny print, my pencil in my hand, my brain drowsy as the docs came in this morning. There was nothing slow or steady about that twenty minutes in my room. Within a minute they had removed my twelve-hour old dressing which was saturated by fluid that continues to drain (not knowing that the "drain" is gone!) The docs did "their list" of stuff to do and meds to take, then it was my turn.

I wanted to know about meds and what to wear and follow up and such. That "what to wear" seemed so odd to have to ask, but this incision is around a foot long....they suggested "boxers'"" rather than "briefs" for a while. Oh, my....

Then I was asking them about my blood levels. I have tracked that a bit because I am a blood donor. Even as I asked him the question, I had the realization that my blood donating days might be done....over with, maybe, because of cancer. I lost it.

I had been so very "professional" right through the Q&A period here this morning in my room ... at that time, it wasn't me, the former nurse, it was just me, who values blood donation....who has cancer....who has one more little thing that is interrupted by a bunch of cells that are so incredibly UN-welcomed in my body.

This step of the main tumor removal has been so important. I want to take more steps...leaps of faith even. Maybe that is why I was crying. What is the next thing to do.... what more is required...who can take this stuff out of my lungs...is it a surgery...who would do it? The docs refocused me to this day, to this recovery, to watching and waiting.

Focus is good. Focus is needed. I have worked on this post 5 times in the past 3 hours because I just can't focus well....tired....meds....low blood pressures...drowsiness.... nausea... bleh.

Jeremiah 29:11 keeps running through my head, *"I know the plans I have for you..."* For me...even me...wrapped in two prayer shawls, watched over by two standing camels, and a Action Figure Jesus, and the ACTUAL Jesus....and a whole bunch of praying saints.

Home Sweet Home
Posted Oct 25, 2011 11:09 p.m.

Home sweet home....with people who would move heaven and earth to help me heal. "Move heaven and earth" = grill salmon, learn to change my dressing, rub my head, back, or legs to distract me and help me relax

31

while the meds take effect, drive home safely, pass the tissues to me when I am overwhelmed and weeping, fetch the prayer shawls, pray over our meal, install a new raised toilet seat with arms. As a person in a great deal of pain and at the end of a long day, I still can't imagine I could be more deeply blessed.

For everything there is a season
Posted Oct 26, 2011 11:53 p.m.

I am all for "seasons" outside. I especially love fall and spring. This fall, I am especially thankful that Dad and Mom are retired as they are a huge help to me in my care.
I am a bit frustrated because of a mix up of "seasons of life." At 50, I didn't anticipate experiencing the joy of an elevated toilet seat, an improvised carry-bag on the front of my borrowed walker, and three concurrent intestinal support medications.
My mind wanders through many areas of thanks, even just sitting up for eight minutes to type is a blessing! What I settle on, though, is that I appreciate the time (96 years and counting) that I have had with my Grandpa Harding...and the time, effort and energy that the folks at St. Francis Hospital are investing in his care....and for the time I had to share my love for him in a letter, that had to "be my voice present in his room" when I couldn't be there myself.
This morning my Bible time went straight to Psalm 23...*The Lord is my shepherd....*
Yep. Because right now, *"Even though I walk through the darkest valley, I will fear no evil, for you are with me; your rod and your staff, they comfort me."*
Grandpa's valley, my valley, my family's valley, the valleys that others are experiencing. For over 26 years I have smiled when I thought of the words "rod and your staff" as my husband Rod, and the people on his staff, because he usually had one. It was many years later that I got the point (literally) that the shepherd's rod would direct me to go this way or that....and the staff with that big hook would pull me back upright when I

32

had fallen and couldn't get up (which isn't beyond the stretch of the imagination today).

I guess I have mixed feelings about this particular time...thankful, worried, hopeful, foggy, overwhelmed, encouraged, sleepy, (repeat until no longer directed...)

I need to spend my time here at home, healing. However, I'll admit that when my heart is divided between here and St. Francis, and Manchester Hall at Illinois State, and the rooms of this house....well...it is complicated. Tonight, I will sleep knowing as truth what Grandma and Grandpa Harding said in that card 23 years ago....and was repeated in the note I sent to Grandpa today.... "We're not so very far apart, God can see us both." Valley or not.

Bit by bit
Posted Oct 28, 2011 12:52 a.m.

A few weeks ago, it was morning time...fresh off breakfast, scripture and prayer, in the recliner with the early fall sunlight streaming in on me that I found my muse....first writing for me, then for others.

Now I'm not so sure how to find that muse again. With the house full of people and my needs for support so great it is hard to set my mind apart to wrestle through some things until late at night.

Earlier today after a nap I sat up and took a deep breath and it hurt....sharp little pains over my lungs, kind of under my arms and radiating to the back. I figured it could help me to use the incentive spirometer (breathing apparatus) that I had used faithfully in the hospital. I tried it and it still hurt. That wore on me through the day. I used some of my nursing knowledge, and a dose of fear, and went down one unhealthy path and up another. By the time I mentioned it to my mom I was tearful. Yes, I would call Eric. He called back later and we figured that the pain had more to do with the muscles I was using "anew" from the walker, than from rampant cell growth out of one of the slowest cancers ever, in my lungs.

33

The day also included a dressing change, which my mom has perfected....with very little drainage (hurray), but this was green! I think this is a long way to go to demonstrate my FROGGINESS....however, it did mean that I needed to make a call to the clinic....and all is OK. The day included odd pain in my left palm...really? So we changed the padding on the walker handle with some awesome Duck Tape, but then right on the creases it hurt even more. We are still working on a solution to that. Just below the center of my palm, it is a bit numb....nerve irritation, I think.

We are still praying through Grandpa Harding's condition, and other things in the lives of our extended family and friends. Bit by bit.
One thing I am learning about me, bit by bit, is something I need to be "me"....I need to sort out life and to lift up the connections between faith and life.....sometimes for me....sometimes for others. In my call at Trinity, I get to do that every day. I love what I do. It is, however, also who I am. God is using you all to help me understand that. I think, that in no small way, by continuing to do this praying and writing and reading that God will remind me of whose I am and who I am (Child of God) every day. And, that through that, I will have hope.

I just got a lovely cross....a non-traditional cross....a Tau cross....that looks a lot like the capital letter "T". When I see that cross I am reminded of the incompleteness of our understanding of God's love and grace. We get to see SO much of it through Jesus, and through the written Word and the preached word and through God's great meal and washing in water....but we don't see it all. I think I would rather see it all. I mean, really! This living day to day....this waiting to heal...using a walker....this always having to have someone with me....this not being able to drive, or think clearly....frustrates me. And, has me afraid. Let's see how this will all play out. I would like control. Really?
Bit by bit....
"For now we see in a mirror dimly; but then face to face: now I know in part; but then shall I know even as also I am known." (1 Cor. 13:12).
Thanks for accepting my continued striving to be whole and well....and still me....

Goals, just a few...
Posted Oct 28, 2011 6:39 p.m.

So, I headed into today with a few goals...I mean really, if I am going to be so darn strong and courageous then I need to be strong and courageous at doing "something," right? And, this whole sort of a "goal for the day" could help me move beyond the "fear-a-day or "period-of-pain" that has seemed to encroach on my regularly scheduled life.

(In case I forget to thank you later....this day was made possible by (1) God; (2) my current in-home caregivers/encouragers.... Mom and Erica; (3) all of you encourager/prayer types....I would hate it if you quit doing what you do so well for lack of affirmation.)

So, back to the goals. I did not have my mom set an alarm to wake me up for pain meds this last morning, just in case we slept well. And, by "we" I meant "me," as I can barely make myself sleep well, let alone take on another human's sleep. Then...in the midst of this goal, another goal was met. I woke up at about 3 a.m., not needing pain meds so much, even though I could have taken more, as much as I needed to go to the bathroom. Some of you know that that great new "elevated throne" is actually in my bedroom, which makes this (plus showering and brushing my teeth pretty convenient. So....after using the throne I returned to bed....to sit on it. Mom did not wake up from my light being on.....she was asleep on the sofa in the living room (done at her own personal sacrifice so she could be in earshot if I needed her in the night). I decided to try to get my legs back up in the bed on my own....(the right leg being the problem child, as it has very little outward lateral movement since the tumor was removed and the muscles all "messed with"). Guess what! I did it! WooHoo! This is huge, people. Nine days of "no ability" replaced with "Woohoo!"

Then, we both slept until 7:30 a.m. This in itself is a goal met for me....no pain meds for eight hours (usually I only go four hours at a time during the day). I must be getting better. Mom vacillated between shock, awe, and "I kept having these dreams about you needing to get up for meds."

Then, this morning, with 1/2 the usual meds I would take, I rested in the recliner or sat in the office chair in the dining room and did NOT return to the bed as per usual on the previous eight days. I also "supervised" the work of a dear friend in Halloween-decorating of the front porch. I am a formidable supervisor in boxers standing with my walker at the front screen door. She did a great job! Some of the camels are now even in costume for trick or treating!

I even found the ability to stand outside in the sunshine on the deck, which is a bit of a logistical challenge with the walker and all, but well worth it. (Thanks to those who suggested it.)

In fact, I did not return to bed until 4 p.m., and maintained a pleasant disposition. Many might not think this a big deal. However, some might think that such things as two surgeries in twenty days or cancer or twelve inches or so of stitches in my right hip could have blown my cool, but no. I had a goal (with Erica). This was the "Afternoon of the Consolidation of the Elder Daughter's College Student Loans." I had done the preliminary work of (1) giving birth; (2) helping select a college; (3) making payments for stuff not covered by grants, scholarships, and loans; (4) keeping files with lots of important papers, and (5) moving her back home after graduation. This was my afternoon to sit still and be a non-anxious-presence as she completed the process to propel her on a 20-year-relationship with a lender. I hung in there through "step 3 of 8 or step 5 of 9 in the electronic signing of the Master Promissory Note. Then, I was....and still remain "toast."

As I returned to bed, I had Erica wait to watch me show off my "I can get to bed on my own" skills, which seem to have waned a bit in the last twelve hours. I made it, but it wasn't pretty. Then as she left the room there was some crack about "differently-abled" which I will ignore.

Goals achieved. Day lived. I am so relieved. I am practically giddy, although not actually having the energy needed to display it.

Oh yes, and I relay this result of a courageous and strong day by 5:30 p.m., well before the Cardinals play in the last game of the World Series. I have many dear friends whom I love and respect who have affection for the Cardinals so I will remain joyful for them. I have confidence that the Cubs' year is coming. I look forward to living to see it. I believe that God still works miracles every day; however I cannot orchestrate it, so the Cubbies are still going to have to practice, and then play games and win them. We all have goals.

Hmmm.... Q & A

Posted Oct 30, 2011 5:49 p.m.

So it seems that along the way, some of you are asking some questions. Here are a few:

(1) Whose Nerf football is it that was left in the back yard after my 50th birthday party?

(Ok, I asked this....but still no claimers....)

(2) Dad asked, "So how is your sciatic pain?"

That question sort of took me aback. I have probably been telling anyone who couldn't out run me about my sciatic pain since last Nov/Dec/Jan. Until 4 p.m., or so, of October 19, it was my #1 or #2 concern (alternating with sarcoma). It is a bit hard to say. After the first week or so from surgery, I don't really recognize much of any pain lower than my knee on my right leg. The pain is really all about my right hip and the surrounds now. Narcotics and Neuronten (for the nerve pain) seem to pretty much take care of my pain....that and not having a tumor a bit larger than a softball in my hip. I seem to have moved on to "what-ever-hurts-me-lately". I am happy to say that my back feels just great, thank you. And I want to publicly apologize to my back for all of the demeaning things I said about it for the last nine months.

(3) How long is the incision, really? (This was my question.)

I made dad get my Alltrade 16 Ft. Tape Measure the last time mom did a dressing change to check. I estimated twelve inches....especially because the original dressing went from my right arm pit to below my knee (just kidding), but it really was over a foot long. So the actual length is just about 9 1/2 inches. (There is a little curve to it, and my calculus is rusty, and I was NOT about to let that tape measure touch those stitches). Dad mentioned that maybe it would be a great start for a tattoo. After a bit of discussion about a tattoo map of route 116 going through Owego Township (where I grew up in Livingston County, IL) , or the Mississippi River etc, I've decided to drop that whole idea.

(4) "Do you need meals?" ....asked by many.

Totally, yes....I think we all do! However, because mom and/or mom & dad are here with us, we really don't need meals delivered. When I get to the time when other folks aren't living here with us that could change.

(5) What is your next "window?"

I am thankful to be moving from the "when is my next pain medication due" series of windows, for sure. I am pretty focused on how I will be decorating my pumpkin for Halloween, so that is a "before 5 p.m. on Monday" window. The bigger window is Tuesday, November 8, when I return for a post-operative visit with my surgeon and a visit with the oncologist. That will be just shy of three weeks from surgery, and right about six weeks from when my first CT with contrast scan revealed the metastases in my lungs. Dr. Mo said that the second scan would be at eight weeks. The cytogenics (genetic testing) done on the tumor sampling in the biopsy surgery did not grow in the lab to show anything at all. We knew that this would be a possibility. I'm not sure if they will repeat this genetic testing on the tumor itself. This could tell us some more about how the tumor works, just in case chemotherapy is needed later.

(6) I wonder how much longer I will have to use this ol' walker? (asked by me) "Keep using it!" (Mom's reply)

I can truly appreciate those folks in the flock who have had to move to a "use-a-walker" life. First, you have to get rid of anything in your path that a walker would not go over or just bunch up...even if it just looks better when those things are there. (e.g., rugs) Then, you have to have a path as wide as the walker -- everywhere. It all could be great, then someone might bring in groceries or a coat or somethin' and ya' have to start over.

Things that help, Part 4
Posted Oct 31, 2011 1:13 p.m.

It is a short, focused list this time, of things that help.
(1) Prayers....keep them coming, including prayers for my grandpa, Roger Harding, who continues to struggle because of pneumonia at St. Francis in Peoria...and for his sons, my dad and Uncle Dennis, who are coordinating his care.
(2) Having a brief craft project. There is no way that I could carve a pumpkin this year. (carving knives + me + my meds = trouble). So this year it is "painting" as decorating.
(3) Matthew 6:25-34....I keep reading and reading.... and the poem *"Sacrament of Letting Go"* by Sister Macrina Wierderkehr, sent to me by a friend who has had recurrent battles with breast cancer. I've been reading this each morning, and through the day. I suggest looking up, and reading both.

Healing, by the numbers
Posted Nov 2, 2011 1:53 p.m.

One good name for us: Children of God. I found this in my reading this morning; 1 John 3:1-3 *"See what love the Father has given us, that we should be called children of God; and that is what we are."*

1... The number of Hoya plants that have decided to bloom yet again (within a two month period!) This is remarkable!
2... The number of weeks ago today that I had surgery. Honestly it amazes me how much progress I have made.
4... The number of beautiful mum plants that I've received lately that are now planted outside
5... How many family members have birthdays in the first 13 days of November -- including daughter Sarah, who turns 19 on November 12!
6... The number of days I have to wait until I head back to Iowa City to see my doctors, get rid of the stitches and such. Thank goodness for those blue wheel chair things there, otherwise I think we might need to head

over in four days, just to give me time to walk from the drop off place to the doctor's office!

6... The number of ideas that folks have given for my hand grips on the walker.

12... The number of Tegaderm dressings that I needed from a medical supply place to get me through until the appointment on November 8. I use three each time the dressing is changed. They cost $4.55 each. Man alive that was some serious rigamarole to get it figured out regarding what insurance covered it. The extremes of the story included "no coverage and a cost of $370" to "85% coverage and a cost of around $8.50." (I truly give thanks for good insurance coverage.)

26... How many individual pills I take a day (15 of them pack some punch!)

75... About how many minutes I was outside yesterday afternoon....it was so so beautiful. I visited with Penny who did the "mum gardening" and emptied the flower pots on the deck, and put the pots in the shed. I even took one step down (!) using the walker, of course, to the larger level of the deck....and used scissors to help trim the plants. It turns out I can do that if I am standing straight, but not so much if I have to bend over. Live and learn.

100... How many trick or treaters we had here at home (FYI, the purple, green and black PlayDoh went first).

500... How many cc's drained from Grandpa's chest tube with the first round of treatment...about 1/4 of what has accumulated in his lungs....keep praying.

Restaurant or "Work-aurant"
Posted Nov 3, 2011 12:24 p.m.

This is the scene: I am in the recliner in the living room. Dad has gone out to the front porch to retrieve the outdoor thermometer, now broken. He installed it several days ago. It was a good purchase, as it allowed all of us to serve in our appointed roles as late-fall meteorologists from the comfort of indoor temperatures. (Those of the "Romper Room" era might appreciate my fascination with meteorology born of my love of the role of Wendy the Weather Girl.)

Late last evening wind blew the thermometer off its bracket, landing on the porch. In the dark, dad replaced the thermometer and went on to bed. Mom and I didn't know all this. This morning, mom (serving as morning meteorologist) went to check the temperature and found that the thermometer, in its "regular position" was broken. This puzzled the two of us. Did Bob, the black squirrel who lives in the front porch pillar to which the thermometer is affixed, get ticked off, and come out and break it? Why would he be angry about the thermometer? He didn't seem to mind other things; for instance the Halloween garland. Or, how could wind break the glass only? So we wondered for about 30 minutes until dad filled us in.

Dad, (a farmer) and the rest of us, were a bit disappointed at this turn of events. I have had this house for over eight years with no outdoor thermometer. Who knows what temperature it might be out there? (Of course there are three computers within a fifteen foot radius of the dining room table in our modest main floor which could tell us that information in a nano-second.) So, dad moves into the project mode of removing the broken thermometer.

As he does this, I see an opportunity to get the Halloween stuff off the porch and start passing instructions about what could come down to dad (who is out on the front porch) via mom (who is inside my noisy antique front door/screen door combination). The instructions come in bits....to include, taking down the Halloween garland, taking down the decorative Halloween cloth that hangs outside, moving the pumpkins to the back porch (for our continued enjoyment), and moving the little table that held a pumpkin to the back patio.

Each of those instructions came after about a ten second pause, during which the doors were closed ....pause...the doors were opened....dad's attention was regained and the new directive was given. After about the third directive dad just started laughing.

Mom's response was "Did you think this was a restaurant? It is a work-aurant!" This cracked us all up.

Perhaps even more funny to me was to hear dad's recollection of the events from his perspective on the porch (once he came back inside). "First I would hear the rustle-rustle of the doors. Then your mom would

41

come out with something for me to do...then she would go....then the rustle-rustle...then the thing to do....then she would go....rustle-rustle....stuff to do..." This cracked me up... It is good to laugh. Yep, after weeks of tears, stress, and sadness, it is good to laugh.

It is also good to have good work. My oh my, I miss work.
I miss just doing stuff....like unloading the dishwasher for heaven's sake! It was some sort of reportable event amongst the family when I helped by emptying a bag of chocolate chips and a cup and a half of peanut butter into a bowl as my mom made Puppy Chow treats.
Yesterday was a "bleh" day. I lacked focus for the stuff I could do sitting down. It seemed like my back, hip, leg all had some little bit of swelling that made it hard to sit. The sciatic pain down my leg returned. It seems like some of the nerves in my hip are "waking up" as mom says. It has been two weeks and a day since surgery and I am mentally ready to participate in the "work-aurant." I remember that Golden Rule to love my neighbor as myself. Surely that means "do something," doesn't it?
I find myself reaching to draw on my sabbatical experience of last summer. It took me the first two of those three months to slow down and really rest. (I do have "work-aurant" in my genes.)

This time it is my *body* as well as my *spirit* that needs healing. I can use some prayer support on this....for focus to let this happen...for patience in this process. I don't have a triple-doppler-radar to help me know what is going on inside my body. If I did, I would have gotten at this fibromxyosarcoma a lot earlier, that is for sure! (Of course, in my mind "working equals being healthy," too.) This healing from the surgery just takes the time it is going to take. (repeat to self....) Breathe. Somehow, this physical, mental and spiritual work is some of the hardest I have ever done. I guess this is a "work-aurant" after all...

Just trying to sort it all out
Posted Nov 5, 2011 12:03 a.m.

Some days, I just feel like I'm trying to sort this all out. A day or two ago (I don't remember) I mentioned how much I longed to return to ministry or something like that. I miss the staff and all the folks at Trinity Lutheran Church so much. However, I do know that I need to pay very close attention to taking the steps I need to protect this time of healing. I won't mess this up. I can't. There isn't any room in my life for "not getting well." However, that isn't what is bugging me. What I can't let rest is the notion that I might be portraying ministry as something that is only done when I "go back to it." I *do* ministry every day...by thanking my parents, by loving my daughters, by praying for you all and myself, by striving for healing, and more. We don't need theological degrees to *do ministry*. Love God. Love your neighbor. I just had to let you know where I stand on that. Now, return to the ministry you all are doing so beautifully...that's it....you can do it...

With all the saints
Posted Nov 5, 2011 7:19 p.m.

Today, my daughters, my family and I remember my husband Rod. He entered eternal life seven years ago this afternoon. I strive to have half the courage he had as he faced cancer. Through his experience, I learned that cancer does not ever win. God wins.

Tomorrow in worship, the saints who entered eternal life, and the saints who became children of God by baptism in this past year will be remembered and embraced. It has been my honor and joy to walk with families experiencing one or the other...and in a few cases both, within this past year. My prayers are with you all.

My reading in the recliner today comes from tomorrow's All Saints Sunday's story from Revelation 7:9-17....which ends, "*...and God will wipe away every tear from their eyes.*" Amen

Still sorting...
Posted Nov 8, 2011 12:45 a.m.

Sunday, I celebrated the Sabbath....only writing for me (not the CarePage) and for God. God and me, sorting.

Today, Monday. Still sorting.

It has been a hard sorting day. It feels like I have developed something akin to "post traumatic stress" regarding going to University of Iowa Hospitals and Clinics. I'll tell ya folks, two runs through the offices of those dear, smart, caring people, with news that felt as far off plum as you can get, can do that to a person, even me.

So, here I have stewed and prayed. I have been changing over to Ibuprofen from Percocet through the morning and early afternoon. This has been pretty smooth. It is nice not to feel so foggy. It is nice to have better balance. (I've even gone about three full days without needing the walker.) One other med still makes me drowsy, but that is just the way it is going to be for a while.

So, I took my stewing, sorting, praying self outside. I sat in a chair on the upper deck. I did a little project in that chair. I prayed. Still sorting and stewing. It looks as though my Grandpa Harding is likely headed to hospice care. I took my non-dizzy self down the 1-plus-3 more steps off the deck to the patio and on to the grass. Usually, just standing on grass somewhere, anywhere can help me re-set my spirit. Slowly I walked and stewed and sorted and prayed.

There are some days in life when even though nothing changes, one knows that something is about to change. The pain of that day in anticipating a change is every bit as much as pain on the day of the change. Today was my pain day for Grandpa. How many women can boast of a 50-plus year relationship with a grandparent-cheerleader-friend? I am blessed beyond measure.

So, what happened for all this stewing, sorting, praying, and even walking outside without my mom even knowing (yikes...)? A few things. I found great comfort knowing Dad was visiting Grandpa today, and that one of their pastors, Rev. Heidi Punt, had brought him communion. And he received it and prayed and knew what was going on in those moments. I have brought that precious meal to more people than I can count. Today I

44

couldn't do that, but the point is God was there with Grandpa. God's love poured out over him with the assurance of the kind of life that we can't promise with modern medicine. I am so thankful.

Tomorrow I return to Iowa City, stress or no stress. These appointments will be about taking out stitches and waiting in waiting rooms to find out what date I am waiting for next! Actually, that I can handle. Stitches and waiting. Stitches and waiting. Dear Lord, please no bad news. Please just stitches and waiting.

The day of stitches and waiting
Posted Nov 8, 2011 6:29 p.m.

That was it in a nutshell. Stitch removal and waiting and waiting and waiting.

So, the stitches go like this. Get up. Ride to the Clinic in Iowa City. Ride in the wheelchair-like contraption to the I-elevator as Erica learns how to use/not-use the brake on said contraption. Erica learns, I crack up... One waiting room. One nurse. One resident. One surgeon with the same resident and one med student...message being....there was a LOT of stuff moved around in there (read "hip") and now there is a fair-sized hematoma (read "an area that is numb about the size of my fist along my incision"). Many empathetic nods. Questions answered, including that there could be microscopic bits of the cancer left in my hip. Surgeon and his squad leave the room and a nurse with two gloves, *sharp* scissors, tweezers, and a blend of speed-all-business-empathy enters. I realized that I need to grip *something*. I choose Erica's hand as she offers it to me. (Later she admits that she offers it in thankfulness for the zillion times I had helped her through "stuff" including injections.)

Fortunately the nurse could "read" my tension to know that I needed a few breaks in the action along the way. Fortunately Erica and Mom and the physician's assistant understood my pleas for distracting conversation so we chatted about what cafeteria to eat at in the hospital. The "stimulating conversation" worked. Oh-My-Goodness! It is fascinating to me that I dreaded that ol' drain removal for days and didn't dread this. Boy did I

45

have that goofed up! So much for my weaning off of Percocet. It is my best friend today. Whew. My next best friend is that ol' wheelchair. Thank the Lord for the wheelchair. I am even back to using the walker at home. Fortunately this should be a short lived setback.

The surgeon waiting is done, and the next waiting goes like this. The oncology waiting room has a puzzle. Mom and I work on that ol" 1000 piece puzzle of a panda bear like we are scientists from the jet propulsion laboratory. One hour later we came up for air when my name was called. More waiting. Then Dr. Mo says my cancer has a new name now that the pathologists have gotten to know it better. Here it is...
Sclerosing epitheloid fibrosarcoma. It means something like "scar-forming-lining-scar-forming-cancer," which is slow growing still and still rare and still needs more waiting.

So, here is the new window. "Two weeks." In two weeks, on November 22, I return for lab tests, a repeat CT scan and appointment with Dr. Mo. Then, when we see that the cancer in my lungs isn't growing at *all* (...prayer request hidden in that), we will continue to watch it and set the next window. It is a little odd to think that my cancer has another name...I had just gotten to know that other name and now feel like I am getting to know a stranger.

Now, I'm home. Supper is ready. Grandpa has been moved for care back to his home town. Tomorrow I may say more about the scripture that seemed to help today as well. But, supper is ready now, and I'm thankful for that.

Sorting and fear, and figuring it out
Posted Nov 9, 2011 8:30 p.m.

Part of my sorting has revealed that I truly expected to be more recovered at three weeks. I've had one other bigger surgery on my shoulder and that did take a long time to heal...hum...but this time, my mobility is affected. And I am frustrated. And sore. And I do have cancer...oh, that's right...

46

So I go back to the thought that came yesterday morning. The thought from that reading of Matthew 25 and the parable of the talents. In a nutshell, the land owner doles out wages to each of three slaves in decreasing amounts, the least of whom receives the equivalent of about fifteen years wages and goes away. Upon return, the first two have increased the investment but the third only returns the original investment that was kept safe in a hole in the ground. The first and second are rewarded. The third is not. This is a great/typical stewardship lesson told by me and countless pastors in "stewardship season" before. But this year, something else captures me. Fear. That third guy fears the land owner. He thinks the land owner is "to-be-feared" amongst many other things, so he just hands back the money he was given. Maybe this is more a parable of relationship. The first two have a wonderful relationship with the landowner (God)....the third, no. It made me stop and think about my relationship with God. I have a good one.

However, it is pretty darn easy for me to set aside that primary relationship, and pick up a fear-filled relationship with my cancer as my primary relationship. I can let it spill over into other stuff like hip/leg pain when I'm still healing from a major-destructive-reconstructive surgery.
It is not wrong to have fear. I still have it. However, I don't need to let it be my "number-one-anything." I cannot begin to describe how difficult this cancer journey is mentally, especially if I apply my imagination to it at all! I might (or probably will) visit "Fear-ville" and "Worry-town" on one trip or another, but I don't have to let them be my destination.

Joys of the day
Posted Nov 10, 2011 8:14 p.m.

A combination of your prayers, the expressing/purging of my current fears to yours and God's caring ears, and better pain control have all helped me move into this better day, which includes these joys:
1) Setting a goal of writing some notes to people and doing that with a new yellow pen in hand
2) Two hours or so with mom who said "yes" she would like a Pinterest account (because I have one and it's cool), and then "yes, ok" to a

Facebook account when we figured out that she couldn't have a Pinterest account unless she was on Facebook or Twitter. Then, to hear mom tell dad about who had "friended her" and "who posted what" was just a hoot.

3) Announcing to my daughters that their Grandma Harding was on Facebook. I am still laughing.

4) Teaching my mom how to change the wall paper on her computer, which now sports a photo that dad took of mom as she had climbed to some height in Arches National Park in Utah.

5) Being able to love and encourage a friend who has also had a recent cancer experience. One thing I have been reminded of in these past eight years of ministry is that whatever we have wrong with us, or whatever loss is experienced, that it is not a "contest" of what hardship is worse than any other hardship. All of us stand in need of care from God and one another. It is my honor to offer the consolation that I have received from God as well. (2 Cor. 1:4)

6) Looking ahead....toward Thanksgiving...what a great holiday to have ahead, for I am thankful. Yes, I am.

Simple things
Posted Nov 11, 2011 11:11 p.m.

Perhaps because some of this journey with sclerosing epitheloid fibrosarcoma is so complex, and because a good portion of my days include a significant amount of soreness that I find that some of the simple things of life are appreciated and become even more beautiful. Today, these things are: leisurely conversations with family after a good meal, "Dancing with the Stars" on TV, and unexpected visits from friends.

The care of sighs
Posted Nov 12, 2011 6:36 p.m.

I can't help but notice my use of "sighs" through the day. Sighs when I am sad or frustrated, tired or sore. A dear pastor friend offered me the gracious image of the One who gathers up those sighs.
That was my meditation this afternoon.

I imagined these many sighs...sighs drifting and swirling low around me...and the Spirit of God bending low and gathering them close to Her chest and holding them there as they are precious to Her. I see the Spirit swirling round the cross of Jesus in his pain as he sighs...and those sighs gathered up and held...inhaled. Is that how it "works" I wonder...? The Spirit inhales our sighs and exhales peace...is that how our burdens are held? Sighs and peace. Sighs and peace. I try it. Offering my sighs....inhaling that peace.... Offering my sighs. Inhaling peace. It feels good. It feels good to think that those bits of cancer in my lungs are surrounded in peace. Slow down...slow down, I say. I try it again. *"The Spirit intercedes for us, with sighs too deep for us to express."* (loosely translated from Romans 8:26) Thanks be to God...

The more I think about this, the less concerned I am that I sigh.... Though perhaps it seems odd to even say that. Of course, what I mind are the very things that I am sighing about....pain, weariness, worry, uncertainly, separation, frustration, impatience, boredom, fear, the cancer.

But this gathering up of my sighs, our sighs...that is beautiful. That is hopeful. The sigh is not the end, it is a part of the conversation of breathing....The Spirit to me. Me to the Spirit.

Things that help...Part 5
Posted Nov 15, 2011 9:31 p.m.

1) Reading and re-reading John 20....from the resurrection through Jesus' resurrection appearances. It includes Jesus showing up through locked doors to see the disciples bring them peace, breathe on them, and give them the Holy Spirit. I guess it just helped to read and re-read the extent that Jesus went to to be with people, right where they were....and still does. I figure the only reason I am vertical through some days, well a lot of the last 50 days or so, is because Jesus just shows up and says "I'll stand here. Go ahead and lean."

2) Starting physical therapy. Now I can't say that I feel better physically yet. I am actually more sore and tired. However, I am so glad to begin taking these steps (literally!) toward my healing and recovery. The care of the physical therapists from their listening ears to their wisdom is appreciated. I am thankful that they are being their best selves.

3) Lemon cheese cake. Today, after taking one bite of my college roommate's daughter's freshly made lemon cheesecake I think I fell in love.

Learning stuff along the way
Posted Nov 16, 2011 11:17 p.m.

1) Using the cane for walking longer distances can make it easier to walk further, however I can see how it could increase my tripping risk, as I seem to "kick the cane" every so often. This will take some practice!
2) The process of just learning about long-term disability coverage in over three hours of phone calls in the past two days is equally as stressful as the cancer in those moments. Certainly the whole thing makes me pray all that much harder (if that is possible) that my recovery continues (quickly please) and that my lungs fill with peace, and not cancer.
3) That even as frustrations come up during the day, I am gifted with family and friends and parishioners and colleagues who offer care through calls and cards and notes and rides and prayers. (2 Cor. 4:8-9 "...*hard pressed on every side, but not crushed....*")

Stretch, then strength
Posted Nov 17, 2011 8:36 p.m.

Today was Physical Therapy #2. I faithfully did the simple assignments between sessions. Stand on one foot for 5-7 seconds then the other the same. Repeat, repeat. Stand with one the heel of the right foot at the big toe of the left foot....stand....then reverse....repeat, repeat. Lie on my left side, knees bent, allow the knee of the right leg to touch the surface of the bed next to the left knee (stretching the hip)....wait.....repeat....repeat. Walk with the cane as needed. Massage the incisional area with the intent of releasing adhesions/breaking down scar tissue in the hip (over time).
My assignments for the coming days aren't too much different. My point for describing these simple (although not at all simple until the last week or so) exercises is to say that what I am doing now is all about stretching...not about strengthening.

This stretching has me thinking about something else though, too, -- about how stretching precedes strengthening. I think about the time in college, graduate school, and seminary when some new thought would come along (most classes, most days) that would stretch my understanding. Sometimes these stretching times were uncomfortable! They especially were when the thing I was learning was something about myself! However, what happened next and thereafter most always meant I was stronger or had some greater knowledge and the strength to use that knowledge.

Dear Lord,
Here we are....stretched and stretching. Watch over us. Stick with us. Encourage us. Grow in us what ever needs growing, and help us do and say the things that will reveal that we have grown stronger, even grown stronger in faith and in love of You. Bring healing and support to all of us sighers and stretchers. Amen

Breaking down, building up...
Posted Nov 18, 2011 6:09 p.m.

I admit that I am frustrated. I feel like I am making progress in some of the little day to day things...ease in moving around the kitchen, better balance, and such. Then right along side I have new "aches and pains" in my hip. Some areas that were numb, are super-really-yikes-not-numb anymore! I guess that as that hematoma breaks down, and moves out, there is just going to be pain.
Yet as those particular pains seem to escalate, so does the care from one person or organization or group or another. Yesterday a bouquet arrived from Illinois Wesleyan University's Theta Pi Chapter of Sigma Theta Tau International Nursing Honor Society. Today, a School of Nursing t-shirt arrived with a lovely note from the School of Nursing.
Some of the wonderful homemade bread that has been prepared for the Thanksgiving Eve Worship Service at Trinity Lutheran showed up on my porch during my nap this afternoon.

Somehow each time I struggle, God uses you all to encourage and support me. Let's see...for every action, there is an equal and opposite reaction...I wonder if Newton also experienced this in a life of faith. This is one of many blessings that come with being a part of the church -- the body of Christ.

And the heavens opened up...
Posted Nov 19, 2011 10:26 p.m.

Just as Jesus comes up from out of the water (that wonderful river water), the heavens open up and God talks. Yep. "This is my Son, my Beloved. Listen to him." (Matt. 3)

Today I seem to be acutely aware of voices that are no less precious than the One that came from the cloud that day, by the river, with Jesus still dripping.

Voice #1 -- A friend prayed for me - a lovely prayer. Right there, in the email. I heard her voice. God said as well -- "listen to her...she's a good prayer."

Voice #2 -- (actually, 2, 3 & 4) Mom called. "We are here at Evenglow Lodge. Do you want to talk to your Grandpa? Your dad went to get his phone because it would be easier for Grandpa to use." YES! I want to talk to Grandpa! Then, Dad called back on his phone. Yes, I'm ready. Then, Grandpa's voice, a little quieter, a little more tired, a little less able to take on the usual topics (rain, crops, Cubs, Bears, daughter-update). Rather, we confirmed we missed one another. I confirmed I was getting better and hoped aloud (WITH MY WHOLE HEART) that I am able to travel to Pontiac and see him at Thanksgiving. What a gift that voice of his is to me.

Voices #3 & #4 (or 5 and 6.) -- the sounds of my daughters...laughing, telling stories of school and friends, and best of all, both being right in my house!

Voice through the day...God's voice saying "Hey...it's ok. You can do this, I'm doing this with you."

Thinking, and breathing
Posted Nov 21, 2011 9:41 p.m.

I've been thinking....
1) That the home-Holy-Communion that Pr. Jeff Clements brought on Sunday was exactly what I needed.
2) That I am thankful for the folks at Trinity Hospital and Genesis-Illini Campus in the radiology departments for working so quickly to get copies of some older chest x-rays ready for me. My doctors in Iowa City are interested in them as a basis of comparison with current studies.
3) That my physical therapy is stretching me, and am looking forward to stronger days because I sure am sore today!
4) That I have meditated each day when I started to sigh over one thing or another....sighing out my worries and inhaling peace....sighs and peace. Then I recognized something. I never, ever, exhaled, without inhaling first. I became aware that I was actually inhaling that peace before I ever sighed. What I have come to realize is another example of God's grace -- ready, free, always preceding my need. God's peace is already here, already breathed for me and there for me to receive.
5) And that, that peace has helped me approach tomorrow.

Tomorrow, Tuesday, November 22, I return to Iowa City. Mom, Dad and Sarah will go with me. I begin the day at 10:30 a.m. with a surgeon check-in. At 1 p.m. I have lab tests and at 1:15 I start my prep for a CT scan of my lungs. At 4 p.m. we all meet with Dr. Mo to review the results and plan my further care. Although I reserve the right to get anxious tomorrow, for today I'm ok. My pre-scan-anxiety has been kept at bay. My post-traumatic-stress response to Iowa City in general seems much less as I approach this trip. Thanks be to God. Honestly, it is a peace that passes all understanding.

Dear Lord I hope it lasts through tomorrow! I am so very ready for some good news.

53

Many sighs...
Posted Nov 22, 2011 10:44 p.m.

First, thank you...
The cancer in my lungs has grown ever so slightly in these last 8 weeks. Each lesion growing by a few millimeters. Surgery for the lung lesions is not possible. However, I qualify for a chemotherapy clinical trial. I will begin that shortly after Thanksgiving. There are many physical tests/examinations that I must take and pass before the chemotherapy begins (e.g., lab tests, echocardiogram, EKG) I will also have a port put in in my upper chest for the chemotherapy. The chemotherapy must be delivered at Iowa City because it is their study. I do not know what drug I will be assigned. Two drugs are possible: one is the "standard of care" and one is a very promising new one. The first can only be taken six times, three weeks apart. The second can be taken indefinitely (every three weeks) if it is effective. My doctor has one patient who has been on that second medication with good results for two years. Sigh....

Except for the times I was sobbing today, I did feel peace. I felt peace in the scan. I felt Christ's peace as a gift. I still do. I feel many other things too. I'm so very thankful that every where I go, Christ is there already.
Tomorrow, we head to Pontiac. Erica, Sarah, and I will get to see my Grandpa Harding. This is good. So good. We will see more of Rod's family at my folks as well. Mom and Dad were incredible support for me today. It will be good to be with them for two days. Sigh....

So, please keep praying...for courage, for my family, for healing, for the things I need but frankly can't even think of to type. Sigh....

54

Many thanks...
Posted Nov 24, 2011 12:34 a.m.

There are only some 40 or so minutes left on the Eve of Thanksgiving. I am at my folks' home in Pontiac with Erica and Sarah.

It is also important for me to write this before we celebrate a national day for thanksgiving, for this ordinary, non-holiday-type-of day revealed to me once again many many people who love me and one another.

I worship God who "took on flesh and dwelt among us." (John 1:14) In that joy, I can close my eyes and remember each person, each embrace, even though many have gone on to their homes and the lights of my folks' house are out but for two. God's embrace is just that close. Just that close. Thanks. Thanks be to God.

Holding it together
Posted Nov 25, 2011 12:57 a.m.

Can you imagine one of those metal apple corer-slicers? The ones that are used by standing up the apple and pressing this tool down and through them to make 6-8 slices with the core cut cleanly in the center. When the tool is removed, the slices fall apart from the core. While it is too late at night for me to think too far through this analogy, I definitely had the emotional sensation of having the sharp, harshness of the news from Tuesday (increasing tumor sizes in the lungs and need for chemotherapy to start) cut right through me and I couldn't hold it together any more.

Today what I needed were hugs. Fortunately my mom and dad were right there when I started to crumble. My grandfather's hugs helped too. Those hugs make me think of those slices of apple that can be held together to the core after being sliced. When the people who love me bear these burdens with me, it makes it possible to remember my core...Christ's presence and love and hope.

Little things...
Posted Nov 25, 2011 11:58 p.m.

Some times "it's the little things" that seem to make a difference. I'll list a few of them here, knowing full well that they are big things to me...
1) Remembering my Grandma Davis, whose ring I wear. In my young adulthood Grandma had breast cancer. In that day folks just didn't talk about cancer. And folks who had breast cancer usually had radical mastectomies. Grandma did. No chemo, no radiation, just a very radical surgery and lengthy recovery. I am so glad there is hope for a cure for people with breast cancer that is not so disfiguring and also offers long life. This morning, the memory of Grandma, brought me a touch point and a lift out of my sadness. Grandma demonstrated the possibility of recovery life against great odds. I am thankful for that woman of great grace and for all my grandparents.
2) My fall yard work is done. The Schultz family and the Johnson family may say their help was a little thing to them but to me, well, you know.
3) Family dinner time with Erica and Sarah. A great blend of food and laughter, memories shared of life at Wartburg Seminary, and living at Grandma Koppenhoefer's house in the summers. And on and on...
4) Chauffer service....today by a a dear friend to physical therapy, lunch and Walgreens drive-through (again)...more than just a drive, the conversation and listening ear as I fill tissues with tears over a single butter burger basket, it was a help to me in body, mind and spirit.
5) A quick reply. Today, with questions swirling in my head about the clinical trial and about different chemotherapy drugs and when to start and how many tests there were, I decided to do what Dr. Mo told me to do -- to ask him! To send him an email rather than stew on it. So, I did. He replied, himself, within an hour. So. In short, on Monday, I will talk to the study coordinating nurse. My chemo start date will be set then. (That is no little thing, of course, but rather, hopefully just the thing.)
6) Your prayers, notes, encouragements. Not just little things to me. Just so you know.
This Sunday, the season of Advent begins. I am reminded that Mary's "yes" was no little thing to me, to us, to the world. The Child to come in the manger was no little change to the world....He is everything.

56

Focus... Focus... Focus...
Posted Nov 26, 2011 12:53 p.m.

I seem to mention my grandparents a lot. They have been so important in my life and still are.

Yet today, I am drawing once again on the love of my parents. I cannot imagine a day of this journey, let alone my life. that their love and prayers haven't sustained me.

I could sit in this recliner a long time and remember story after story. Those are good memories. Good areas of focus. Today I printed out Philippians 4:4-9 and posted it in my bathroom mirror. It is a good "touch point" when I lose my focus.

Now, I am going to get ready to make Pumpkin Spice Springerle with my friend Penny. I have a new cookie mold of the life of Christ with sixteen cookies in it. It is lovely. It tells the best story in the world....the one my parents helped me to know. Thank you. Thank you...mom and dad.

Advent hope
Posted Nov 28, 2011 1:13 a.m.

When I got ready for each of the two surgeries, I was completely confident that the doctors, the nurses and all involved would be able to do just what I hoped them to be able to do. And, they did. My tumor named. My tumor removed.

Then, when I found out that the tumors in my lungs were growing (I know...go figure...I thought they were supposed to be SLOW growing) I just crumbled. However, something has been missing -- my confidence in the chemotherapy. This is frustrating. I think Dr. Mo is one of the brightest people I have ever met -- ever. My folks agree. He is also a very caring person. That is a great combination. I have NO doubt that the oncology nurses I meet will be remarkable.

Yet....The days since last Tuesday have taken some paths, mentally, that don't lead toward my full recovery. All that, and I haven't even STARTED the chemo. Oh bother.

But today....today, something happened. Advent happened. Advent is a season *of* waiting. And, it is a season of hope. It is a season of waiting for the absolute best gift ever *and* knowing you already have that gift.

So. I choose hope. I choose to let the doctors and nurses use the absolute best selves they've got on me. I choose to be in a clinical trial so that I have the opportunity to get great meds *and* because I am also a teacher at heart and a life long learner. I want with my whole heart to be well *and* want good to come of all this. I want the next mom, or dad, or sister, or best friend, or neighbor, or neighbor's pastor who gets this ridiculous disease to say, "Hey! No problem! They have *just* the medicine for that!" That is, until the day they say cancer is no more.

More waiting...and hoping
Posted Nov 28, 2011 6:54 p.m.

So, I've learned a few things today.
1) The clinical trial nurse coordinator is great. I told her I would like to start this week. She is working on scheduling the many tests I need, as well as my port insertion, insurance approval, and chemo starting.
2) I can drive. It went fine at the noon hour for eating with friends (even if I did have to get up twice during the meal to walk off some hip pain). However, I learned that just because I *can* drive, doesn't mean that I *have* to. I did a brief trip to HyVee, learning all the way that mid afternoon is way too late in my "pain day" to be doing anything where my hip has to sit right next to the seat belt clip and where I have to walk around much at all.
3) I can wait. Yep. I can. And I am still full of hope. (and a little tired... :)

A hope-filled plan
Posted Nov 29, 2011 6:07 p.m.

So, back to the hope. Hope looks like a facility that has top rated people in the nation, with equipment and technology all in one big place; a clinical trial with access to medications that are available in no other way; access to this facility that is only a little over an hour from my home;

58

people who will advocate for me with my insurance company, and no one at any step has assumed the right to tell me what to do. Rather, they have given me the opportunity to make decisions in my care. With things changing in my body that "have not *ever* asked my permission," I can safely say that that last piece is priceless. I am looking after my own pastoral care needs too, here in town and when in Iowa City from Rev. Cindy Breed, a very dear ELCA chaplain who seems to show up just when I need her.

So, how hopeful am I? My hope is everywhere....like glitter and glue on a preschool project, like lasagna in my refrigerator, like leaves in the ravines, (or in your yard still?) like snow that is hanging out there somewhere just waiting to arrive around here....and like God's love, for there is no place that God is not.

Gifts along the way
Posted Nov 30, 2011 1:52 p.m.

So now that I know when chemo will likely begin, I am thinking about my preparations for Christmas gift giving and am trying to do some now, in case I feel lousy later. However, as I did so, I thought about two gifts I received in the last twelve hours.

1) This gift involves a few things... the prayers of me and others that I would be able to sleep at night again, and the question "Have you read the book *Disrupted: On Fighting Death & Keeping Faith* by Julie Anderson Love, a pastor who survived an extremely malignant brain tumor?" I had not. I ordered it two weeks ago and started reading it....it is amazing. Last night, I read more of it -- maybe for a half hour or so. Then, drowsy and covered by prayer, I slept. Whew. That is a relief.

2) This is about my chemo port. I was offered two choices: regular port which is round, nondescript, doesn't show "too much" when inserted under the skin of the upper chest, *or* a power port, which is a little bit larger, might show a bit more, but can be used not only for chemo and blood draws, but also for the contrast dyes for the many scans in my future. I had quickly picked the regular port. However, a day or two later, I got to thinking. I had chosen my port based on my own sense of heebie jeebies (aka, big versus small...and knowing that it will be inserted under

local...honestly, *local* anesthetic). Sigh. That is not a good way to make that decision. I asked for more information about the ports (aka web site with pictures). These were in my inbox this morning.

Regular port...round, nondescript. Truly it could be the size of a can of tuna but I absolutely know that it is not. Power port....ready for this?! It is pretty! It is amethyst colored. (Which happens to be Rod's birthstone color.) AND it is triangular. Hello! Trinity! God! This is a "no-brainer,"or actually a well-thought-out-prayed-over-choice. I chose the power port. Done. It is perfect. I feel good about it. Oh, what a gift.

Now, when the differences were lifted up to my adult daughter this morning, the response was something like "Mom, you see religious symbolism in everything." Perhaps. But I also see God...sweetly, gently, at work...making what is so scary to me be something that can remind me that God is right here...right in, with, and under me.

Tired...
Posted Dec 1, 2011 11:13 p.m.

As I melt into the recliner tonight I think that a good night's sleep is ahead. Today was the day of Iowa City tests. Except for a few "sticks" (labs and an IV) there wasn't anything painful about the day. Well....I take that back, Mom, Dad and I tried a scone at lunch time that was lacking.
Tonight my "Psalm to sleep with" is 121. *"I lift up my eyes to the hills....from where is my help to come? My help comes from the Lord, the maker of heaven and earth..."* This is a 24/7/365 God. Whew. This is good. Good for us all...for all the world.

Other observations from the recliner
Posted Dec 3, 2011 11:02 p.m.

I see one of the most lovely artificial trees. Ever. Last night as Erica placed the star on the top she asked if I would play "O Christmas Tree" on the piano...which I did, and she offered an interesting re-write of that traditional song to include the closing words "...your leaves are ar-ti-fi-cial." (Pause to try this...)

I see my collection of church ornaments from my family, plus the tiny olive wood nativity that I brought back from Bethlehem. All of them reminding me of places where the coming Child have been seen and heard and loved.

I see the nativity set, the one I received from my Grandma Davis many years ago, on the piano. The baby is tucked safely away in a drawer. That is my personal discipline, which I have enforced in our home....there has to be something besides gifts that arrive on Christmas morning. The baby comes then too.

I see ornaments on our tree. Rod and I gave an ornament to the girls each year, and I continue this tradition. Both of the girls know that my favorite ornaments are the ones from around preschool ages with their pictures in them. I treasured those years and every one since. I couldn't love these two girls more if I tried.

Sometimes I'll hear someone "wonder aloud" if God was/is asleep at the wheel because of my cancer or this disaster or that one. I don't subscribe to that thinking, even if some days God and I wrestle over one thing or another. When that wrestling match is over, God says "Hey, have you seen my Christmas tree....I have the most wonderful pictures of you (and you and you) on it....I couldn't love you (and you and you) more if I tried."

"Amen, I'm alive"
Posted Dec 5, 2011 11:23 a.m.

My title here is from the chorus of the Nickelback song "If Anyone Cared." Their video features the work of some amazing people in contemporary history, around the world, who have cared, and have made major differences in the world.

I am living and hoping and waiting....waiting for Jesus, born to us anew, and waiting for that call from University of Iowa Hospitals and Clinics. This call will tell me which chemo group I am in and what day that will start. Regardless of the content of that call, my wait for Jesus is not in vain. Amen. I'm alive.

Worship and Weeping
Posted Dec 6, 2011 1:22 a.m.

This is about worship. This is about me *in* worship. This is about me missing worship more than I can ever even hope to describe.

In these last two weeks I have been able to get out for one short outing a day. It has certainly improved my quality of life and helped me get a little bit of stamina back. I have to keep the distances I have to walk pretty short. But truly, what I miss is worship. Yes, I miss leading worship and I miss preaching, but I just miss worship.

It was easier to miss worship when I was so medicated that I wasn't so sure what day it was or when I cried each time I got back in my hospital bed.

As I started to feel better, I started worrying about going to worship. I was afraid I would do nothing other than cry during the whole worship service. In fact, as I went to my friend's church, I went to the early service for two reasons...so I wouldn't be around so many people because of potential germs and so I wouldn't see so many people I knew. When I see folks I know, I tend to see them "seeing me," and think I will cry.

Yet. I needed to be there. I got up early. I took my medications early.

Off I went. Cane in hand. Tissues in my pockets. Of course I teared up when I saw my preaching-friend come out to offer the announcements. But I stuck it out. I learned that I needed to sing again. Of course figuring that out made me start crying by the third stanza of the first hymn, but that is why we sing together in worship. Sometimes we are needed to carry the song for one another. That singing was increasingly important. I felt like I was giving my lungs a message "If you are going to grow that *&$#% in there, I am going to fill you with air that is used for praising God! So there!"

Of course, I needed to hear God's surprising call and challenge in preaching. I was not disappointed. Thanks be to God.

But also, I needed to give thanks. Sure I can and do give thanks at home. Every day I do. But I needed to do that in worship. I've been meditating on that section of Phil. 4:6-7 *"Do not worry about anything, but in everything by prayer and supplication with thanksgiving let your requests be made known to God. And the peace of God, which surpasses all understanding,*

62

will guard your hearts and your minds in Christ Jesus." That "with thanksgiving" piece needed me to be in worship....worship is my best thanksgiving....it embodies thanksgiving....the standing and sitting, the listening and speaking, the praying and passing the peace and offering, the tasting and seeing, the confessing and professing, the singing...yes, the singing....all in community, because it is never between just me and God, anyway. Not the community that I have been a part of for the last eight years, but a lovely part of the body of Christ that welcomed me and my few tears this last Sunday morning.

Delight in the ordinary
Posted Dec 6, 2011 11:07 p.m.

Perhaps the key to waiting today was to keep it simple....delight in the ordinary...rejoice in small gains.

I like ordinary days. Simple cooking. Warm laundry on my lap (especially when I didn't do the washing or "flipping" to the dryer). Visiting with my daughters (in person or via text). Sleeping on my stomach. Reading the Isaiah 61 passages for Advent 3. Going up and down stairs three times (albeit slowly). Visiting with friends on the phone. Scrambled eggs with ham and cheese...and fresh-delivered-sweet-rolls. Hearing wonderful music. Not falling in the snow. Working on the Christmas present list for my family.

Each one of these brought some delight. Not just these, of course, but these for sure. Was there "yucky stuff" today? Sure, but I strive to fix my eyes on these things....thankful for the joy of this day. A wise brother in Christ says "Today is a gift. That's why it's called the present." This is true.

Tomorrow will bring new delights. I will look for them. It will also bring news of my next steps.

And the (randomized) winner is...
Posted Dec 7, 2011 6:03 p.m.

Me! So....after a day of ordinary stuff and a lot of waiting the result is:

1) God is good. I pray that this is the chemotherapy that will do the healing. I am thankful for the opportunity to be in this study.

2) I will be receiving Trabectedin (the study drug) given over a 24 hour period every three weeks. (This drug is already approved for use in Europe, and has been for many years.)

3) I will not lose my hair.

4) I will tour the Clinical Research Unit (where I will be receiving the chemo) to get a look at it tomorrow.

5) I will not start the chemotherapy until *next* Tuesday or Thursday. There is no "room in the inn" tomorrow, and they do not do inpatient chemo on Fridays.

6) I still report to the Hospital for my amethyst-colored-triune-shaped Power Port tomorrow morning at 7 a.m. I am hoping for some sleep tonight...and will cherish one more night of tummy-sleeping!

I have seen...
Posted Dec 8, 2011 6:11 p.m.

John 20:29 *Then Jesus told him, "Because you have seen me, you have believed; blessed are those who have not seen and yet have believed."*

Today I saw:

1) a brand new cardiac intervention unit and a brand new cancer center at Iowa City.

2) some amazing nurses and a wonderful resident, all who made me very comfortable, even more so after I admitted my apprehension.

3) once again, the impact of the prayers of *so many* people as I had virtually *no* pain during my amethyst-colored-triune-shaped-power-port use today. And, yes, I was awake for the whole thing! Go figure.

4) My folks accompanying me every step of the way....they are such a blessing...and full of funny stories which always help me.

5) Erica in a surprise morning greeting. Even though I was up at 4:30 a.m., she was up at 5:30, even when she didn't need to be.

6) Judy, the chemotherapy study nurse, escorting me and my folks through the hospital, so that I could see and feel more comfortable with where my chemo will begin *next Tuesday*....arriving there at 8 a.m. and done by about 10 a.m. the next day.

7) Sarah's "check in" with her mom... and, as if she started a flood, there were countless texts, emails, notes on my update, Facebook likes/messages to encourage me and rejoice with me regarding my "good" chemo randomization, and port-day.

8) Two incisions on me...a small one on my right lower neck, and one a little over an inch in length on my right chest, right below that Power Port. I see them and I see hope. This soreness of a few days is *so* worth it for the opportunity to heal and I am thankful.

Jesus talked to those guys who had "seen it all" (in and with Jesus), and he saw that they believed. Then he said that the "blessed ones" will be those who haven't had the privilege but still believe. Granted I live "now" instead of "back then," but certainly I feel blessed to see Jesus at work all over the place. These are just a few of the places I "saw" him today, already!

I have seen, the update.
Posted Dec 8, 2011 6:51 p.m.

Lest you think that post-operative time is all sunshine and puppies...
I am sore.I am grumpy about the soreness.I am grumpy about Erica wearing my favorite socks.I am still sore.

No denying...
Posted Dec 9, 2011 8:53 p.m.

This was my revolution....or perhaps, my evolution, from early this morning....

I am up and dressed (no shower today as the incisions can't get wet until tomorrow) with clean soft clothes. Erica is off to work. The house is quiet. I am waiting for my pain meds to kick in.

I did not think of the port being over my upper ribs. I guess that gives them something to "push against" when the hub needle is inserted. I didn't think of the 3-4 inches of tubing that would run under my skin from the port on to the insertion site in the vein up by my lower neck. That is a pretty darn sore spot. I did not think of how I would be impacted by this "visible sign" of my cancer treatment as I look in the mirror. Before, it was the doctor's computer that held the "cancer" pictures....not my mirror.

Even after the surgeries, the physical therapy, the doctor's appointments, the medications, the "being away" from work at church and all that went with these things, somehow, this morning, I am faced with my former denial of this cancer. That cancer that I can no longer deny.

This morning, as I read from my "Feasting on the Word" preaching resource, the image lifted up by the writer was of a painting by Matthias Grunewold from the 1500s -- Jesus on the cross and John the Baptist/Witness pointing to him. I guess that is what brings me hope this morning...regardless of this cancer or my denial of it, Christ has not denied me, nor will he ever. Thanks be to God.

Things that help, Part 6
Posted Dec 10, 2011 10:57 a.m.

1) Computers and the internet (most of my family should be thankful as well, because this is how I am shopping for their Christmas presents!)
2) New, very soft pajamas -- because these feel so good on the port incisions
3) The season of Advent -- because it helps me "frame" my waiting for healing or tests or whatever, with waiting for the coming of Christ...all other waiting has hope because of this larger lovely loving live-giving gift.
4) Tomorrow's (Sunday, December 11) FUNdraiser for me, held at Trinity Lutheran Church. My dear friend Penny told me her rationale for organizing this FUNdraiser was to have an event to let family and friends

and parishioners put their love into action. It seems like that is the Gospel message: *"Love one another, as I have loved you."* John 13:34.

Two weeks or so ago, I was very disappointed that I couldn't start chemotherapy *that minute*, because the CT scan showed that the cancer was very slowly growing in my lungs. I completed tests, I've had my port insertion, and now await chemo starting on December 13. Sigh. However, this means that if I continue to heal today as I have yesterday, that I will be able to go to the FUNdraiser....to receive the love, freely given, by so many. My oh my....I am already overwhelmed.

Joy
Posted Dec 11, 2011 11:05 p.m.

I am home from the FUNdraiser...after a full evening of talking with so many people -- family, friends, parishioners, community members -- frankly, I find myself speechless.
This is the day that the Lord has made; let us rejoice and be glad in it. Psalm 118:24
This Sunday is Gaudete Sunday -- *to rejoice*, in Latin -- the Third Sunday of Advent. Who knew, that in the middle of such striving, I would find such joy....
The community created and gathered for this event (and the many who were there in spirit) are nothing other than a gift from God....*and* a gracious part of my healing.

Yesterday and tomorrow
Posted Dec 12, 2011 11:11 p.m.

Yesterday was the FUNdraiser....and now, 24 hours later, I am still speechless. Today I learned that over 500 people came. My dad guessed that I greeted only 10-20% of them. I learned that last night alone over $14,000 was raised. This is added to funds that came in ahead of the event and those that came in still today. I am so humbled and thankful for this outpouring of love and care.

Tomorrow, chemotherapy begins. I'll take with me a cd of pictures to look at from the event (I'll get to see all the folks that I didn't get to talk to!). I'll take with me a whole stack of little yellow slips of paper with notes from dozens of people who were at the event last night....I'm saving them all, like doses of love to add to the chemotherapy medication that I will be on from roughly 10 a.m. Tuesday to 10 a.m. Wednesday. *For everything there is a season,* we remember from Ecclesiastes 3:1. Tomorrow begins the season to conquer cancer.....I do this, and I ask God to help and guide me, my doctors, and nurses.

I've got peace
Posted Dec 13, 2011 9:59 p.m.

I keep singing songs of peace in my head today. I have it. I just do. I've had it all day. From bed to shower, home to Iowa City (perhaps except for the I-80 traffic!), main entrance to Clinical Research Unit, exam from Dr. Mo to chemo starting....and now for the first 10 hours of the 24-hour infusion.
Family have been great support, and Mom is staying the night. Anti-nausea meds are working and the "accessing" of the chemo therapy port truly was a breeze (I can't actually believe I am saying that!)
I really have peace about this chemo experience, the medication, my doctor and caregivers. And, truly, a chemo does not have to make me feel *horrible* to work....the new chemotherapies (like this clinical trial med) are especially important to try as they are easier on the healthy part of bodies while they are hard on cancer. I say....thanks be to God, *and let it be so for me according to God's will* (Luke 1:38) (for the curious, I'm "channeling" my inner "Mary" as we approach the 4th Sunday in Advent.)
I can only say that this peace passes all of my understanding.

Peace, and a few aches and pains
Posted Dec 14, 2011 11:03 a.m.

Today comes after a night with not much sleep, a little nausea,, some aches, a headache. All par for the course. I am working on my water consumption....and pretty much am where my doctor says I need to be with 1 gallon a day. (Basically 8 oz. every hour I am awake....16 of them).
I mention this detail here as I know that this big, loving, grace-filled group of "mat carriers" are *prayers* as well as "carriers." Those prayers are precious to me and a huge part of my peace of mind, heart, body, and spirit.
So. This morning, know that the grace poured out, from God and you all, is appreciated beyond measure.

Laura, home...
Posted Dec 14, 2011 10:48 p.m.

Yep, home feels so so good. My chemo lasted about an hour or so more than I expected, but that is okay, as I wanted every precious drop of that medicine!
As I told Mom while at the hospital, if chemo runs a spectrum from "near death" to "puppies and sunshine," then I am way closer to "puppies and sunshine." Thanks be to God.
Tonight, the gift is home...home with both of my daughters...and home with God as well...yep, the God who chose to make a home with us....come Lord Jesus....be our guest...

Nothing is impossible with God
Posted Dec 15, 2011 11:32am

The Luke (chapter 1) story of the annunciation to Mary is one of my favorite in all scripture. Mary speaks, *"Here I am, the servant of the Lord. Let it be with me, according to your word."* I vividly remember being at the Church of the Annunciation in Nazareth. As I entered, I began to weep....and cried all through it....only stopping when I left and walked away to the next site. That church was full of water for me...from me.

Today, I hear the words of Gabriel to the young Mary -- *"Nothing is impossible with God."* Nothing is impossible with God. Nothing is impossible with God. Nothing is impossible with God. I need these Advent words. I pray them like water. I splash them on my head, not worrying if it messes up my hair. I let them soak in. I drink them in. I drink them with the 128 ounces of water I need every day..... Nothing is impossible with God. I sit here, nauseated and tired, floating on these words....buoyed up like I was when I floated on the Dead Sea 18 months ago. I remember that floating...all it required was total release...that's all...just trusting the water to hold me up. That's all. Trusting the water of baptism to be what it is -- God's loving being -- on me, in me, holding me up, making me "me, Child of God" ...even still today. Nothing is impossible with God.

Nausea
Posted Dec 16, 2011 11:20 a.m.
The "sunshine and puppies" phase of this chemo is WAY over with. Remind me again that nothing is impossible with God.

A vigil from afar....
Posted Dec 17, 2011 6:12 p.m.
I'm tethered.

First, I am tethered to this nausea. I have for most of the day just out-nudged the nausea in a winner-take-all contest. I am so determined to win this one. I have three meds and a pair of Sea-bands....and a comfy bed. I will win. (I plan on winning tomorrow, too, but it doesn't know that yet.)

Second, I am tethered to my grandpa....Roger Harding. He is surrounded by my Dad and Mom, by my Uncle Dennis and Aunt Pam, and his pastors all through this day....this precious day. He and I are attached, you see, by some sweet life-long-loving-connection. The wonderful thing is that I get to stay tethered, whether in this life or the next. Whether alive in this life or not, we are both "in Christ." We are both in God's spacious and intimate embrace, one cannot get closer than that.

Of course, I wish that my tethering to nausea was at a much further distance. I wish that my tethering to my grandpa...especially on this day, was much closer. It is hard to be two hours away. Yet, he heard my voice earlier today. Sometime soon he will hear the hosts of angels and Christ's voice of sweet welcome.

Still tethered, to heaven
Posted Dec 19, 2011 11:02 a.m.

Grandpa Harding died early this morning, Monday, December 19, 2011 at age 96 and 1/3 years. My parents and Uncle Dennis and Aunt Pam, and then as of yesterday, his sister Marge, had rotating vigil of him since Friday, a vigil shared in spirit at a distance by his four grandchildren and eight great grandchildren. Honestly, I can't imagine being more blessed than to have had him and my other grandparents in my life.
I sit in the recliner, looking at the Christmas tree that bears two Christmas garland strands....1x1x1/4 inch red, green and gold foil wrapped presents, on a garland strand of long and short gold beads. It hung on Grandma and Grandpa Harding's Christmas trees for as long as they had trees. It has hung on ours for the years since. This morning it looks to me like it holds the whole tree together...every other ornament possible because of that garland that came before it.
Truly though, the garland, the tree, and the gifts collecting around it are only significant because of the One gift that came before us all.

Oh so hoping....
Posted Dec 20, 2011 9:13 p.m.

I am oh so hoping to feel better soon. According to Dr. Mo, I really should not be experiencing any more symptoms from my chemotherapy (aside from taste changes and fatigue). However, something is up. It is a bit of a "perfect storm" of
1) too-long-on-a-lot-of-ibuprofen
2) stress (go figure)
3) dueling anti-nausea arsenal

71

4) wake-me-up-in-the-night nausea pain

5) some more stress

6) pre-chemo med with stomach irritating effects

So....the long and short is this:

    1) call or email Dr. Mo when I feel lousy (there is *no* reason to feel
lousy)-- and I have to tell him how I feel.

    2) drink more water (which will be easier if I don't feel so so bad)

    3) switch meds

    4) I *can* feel better (This feeling better hasn't happened yet, but certainly
I am motivated!)

One of the many gifts of a life of faith, as I know it, is the gift of eternal
life -- life eternally with God, which my grandpa already enjoys, and also
life lived right now to the fullest, whole and well in praise of God. I am so
thankful to be in this clinical trial...and for Dr. Mo's help....now let's get on
with the living!

So very...
Posted Dec 22, 2011 9:56 p.m.

~ thankful, for Grandpa Harding, and the wonderful way he was his "best
self" for our family,

~ in awe of the many people who gathered to give thanks for Grandpa,
who are also a "Livingston County: Pontiac Edition" of a prayer chain for
me and those who care for me,

~ grateful for Dr. Mo who has been checking in on me about every 12
hours to see if I'm getting any better and offering direction for my care

~ grateful for worship today...and the opportunity to feast on the Lord's
Supper, knowing Grandpa gets the whole feast already,

~ thankful for other family members who share my good humor about my
pink-roses-walking-cane (I didn't fall over at all...)

~ looking forward to being on the other side of "wrapping presents,"

~ looking forward to being on the other side of the last few questions on
the long term disability paperwork,

~ looking forward to a good night's sleep,

~ thankful for people who accept Christmas cards in the "spirit" for which they are intended, especially if the season ends up looking more like Ground Hog's Day,

~ thankful for Sarah's driving in these last two days...even through the *snow* on I-39 today,

~ glad that it looks like everything ordered on-line has resulted in in-home delivery,

~ thankful that that one morning, when the women looked inside the tomb, and saw it was empty, and greeted the "gardener" who turned out to be Jesus, that they took their job as the first apostles seriously....and that wise people have continued sharing that good news....even today, with thanks to Rev. Heidi Punt and Rev. Dieter Punt.

This bright cold morning...
Posted Dec 24, 2011 10:30 a.m.

I'm wondering about the shepherds. So much land. So many sheep. Such a big sky. Why hope? Only because God says so. Then this ... an announcement to them, for the world. "Let's go see. If it's so great, then that's it....best news ever. If not, well, we've got the sheep and the land and the sky." But then, just like those angels said, they got it all.
I cast my lot with the shepherds. I have enough. My family. Jesus. Friends. God's promise is enough, but hey, if this hope thing works out...that's everything, yes, that's more than a plenty.
Praying big skies, clear nights, and loved ones near by -- nothing in the way to keep you from hearing the best Good News, nothing in the way to keep you from worshiping the new born King.

I hope...
Posted Dec 27, 2011 12:55 a.m.

Here it is, after Christmas Day by almost a full day. These are some things I hope:
1) That the laughter coming from the living room from my daughters as they play Wii together continues each day. It is good medicine for us all.

2) That I can sort through the "long-term-ness" of this cancer. My mind is more regularly set to a "season" (aka Advent, Christmas, Epiphany) or a short-term-situation (aka, surgery, heal, physical therapy, all better). Somehow as my "knowing about it" reaches three months, I am really ready to just get better and feel better. Sigh.

3) That I can continue to tweak the medicine after chemo to dodge-the-nausea-ball. I do know that life with a water glass in one hand and apple slices in the other can be done.

4) That I never forget the joy of seeing my two little nieces on Christmas morning as they first saw and enjoyed the Barbie Townhouse and groovy Camper! What a hoot.

5) That we always keep telling good Grandpa Harding stories....like each spring when he would get my brother and me new kites and take us kite flying on the country road between our houses. (Do any of you remember how windy it is on a farm?)

6) I will remember how wonderful it was to worship with my daughters, brother and family and parents in celebrating Grandpa's life together, and worship again on Christmas Eve.

7) That people will know my thankfulness for the amazing, encouraging and thoughtful work on the FUNdraiser, whose monetary total is over $20,000, and love and care are priceless.

8) That when I go for labs on Thursday of this week that it will show that my liver is recovering from the first chemo.

9) That my house stays at least as clean as it is now for a while...thanks be to God for helpful daughters!

10) That those of you who are grieving, know God's presence, and of my prayers for comfort. The Christ child is still in the manger, but he has a world of hope for us all. (I just had an image of baby Jesus "thinking," "I would give them all a big hug if I could JUST GET MY HANDS AND ARMS OUT OF THESE SILLY SWADDLING CLOTHES!"

More hoping...
Posted Dec 28, 2011 7:16 p.m.

~ That Sarah gets over the flu FAST -- for her sake and ours as well....this has been a lousy 14 hours so far for her.
~ That Erica and I don't get the flu!
~ That the whole "lab experience" tomorrow (travel, accessing the port, visits with nurse and doctor, and results) are *good* and go well! (The labs are done on Thursday this week because the unit was closed on Monday and Tuesday for the holiday. I don't have any inkling that chemo will be post-poned because of a similar schedule next week.)
~ That the Spirit continues to gather up my "sighs" as She has all along....and breaths back "peace." (I would even take a "side" of patience with that peace.)
~ That my prayers of thanksgiving can exceed my "I needs"

At last...good news, and breathing
Posted Dec 29, 2011 8:05 p.m.

So I figure I can write now...I've been to Iowa City and back with a girlfriend....The blood was drawn (a little difficulty with the port flowing but then, it did). The *long* wait for the labs (about two hours), and then...the *good* news that my liver is recovering! (e.g., one number had been in the mid-200s that came all the way down to 60 today, on the way to a "normal" of 30 or so by next Tuesday as a goal). I told of my "flu" concerns at home and Judy the Research Nurse was very encouraging and affirmed my good-nurse-self-care-flu-prevention-habits. We talked some about chemo for Tuesday, January 3, which looks right on target. Erica and Sarah will accompany me on that trip. Now, seeing Sarah recovering at home, and fixin' to eat leftovers from a wonderful meal that Erica made last night, I'm done sobbing. Yep. Sobbing. Who knew that I was holding my breath? Who knew that I was that worried about today? I feel like I have been given the most spectacular gift on this fifth day of Christmas. I can close my eyes and say with certainty that *this* is what grace "feels" like.

Still with the hope...
Posted Dec 30, 2011 10:49 p.m.

From Lamentations 3.....*But this I call to mind, and therefore I have hope; The steadfast love of the LORD never ceases; His mercies never come to an end; they are new every morning; great is your faithfulness.*

Just like Advent was a good time for me to focus my waiting, Christmas is a wonderful time to focus my hope. I look around my living room and see the Baby Jesus in each manger scene...this is our hope; God with us.
That manger isn't the only location of hope, though. When I came home from Iowa City with good news yesterday, I was reminded that that is a location of hope as well. I have to admit that when time after time I got lousy news, it has been harder to focus on that place as a place of hope. But I remember sitting with Dr. Mo and Judy the Nurse Researcher two visits ago.....weeping my concerns to them and feeling so very sick. Dr. Mo asked why I hadn't let him know it had been so very hard. I'm not sure. I guess I just thought I was doing everything I could do with what I had. He is so very committed to providing excellent care...and if I don't let him know how I am feeling, he can't do that.

I know that Iowa City is a place of hope for me. Now that I feel a bit better, it is physically easier for me to focus on the hope there (although the food part of the inpatient experience is still "colored" by nausea).

My prayer as this year ends and the next begins is for hope. Hope present, waking from sleep in the manger and wiggling loose of swaddling clothes...present here in the living room....present in Iowa City....and at home in the world.

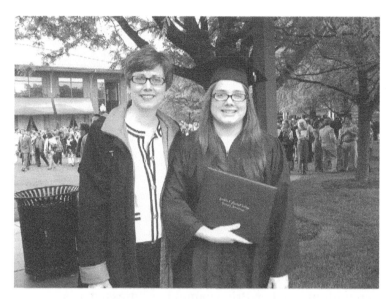

May, 2011-A proud day, as Erica graduates from Franklin & Marshall College in Lancaster, Pennsylvania

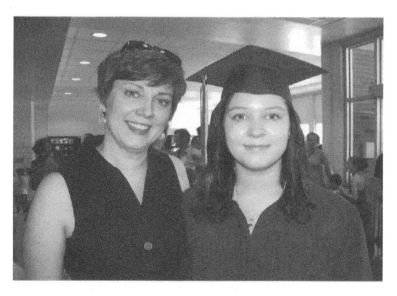

June, 2011 - Another proud day, as Sarah graduates from Rock Island High School in Rock Island, Illinois.

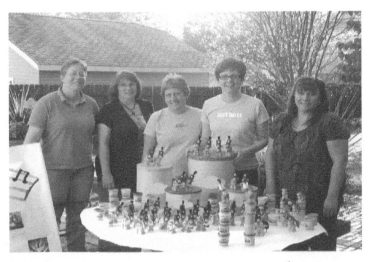

October 5, 2011 - Four friends make my 50th Birthday fun with my Fisher-Price camel herd dressed as a marching band. L to R: Mary Brodd, Nancy Greenwood, Penny Logan, Laura Koppenhoefer, and Becky Wolking.

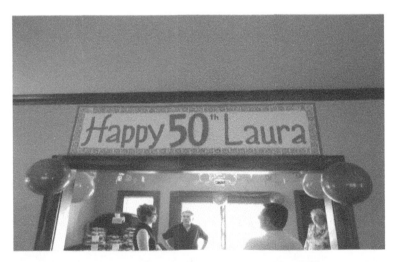

October 8, 2011- A little glimpse of family & friends from near and far in our home. L to R: Laura Koppenhoefer, Steve Koppenhoefer, Tim Kelly, and Sue Koppenhoefer.

2012 UPDATES

New Year...still thankful
Posted Jan 1, 2012 11:22 p.m.

In my bedroom, I have three signs that I received as a gift many years ago. They are three words. Simple words. I've had them surrounding me -- with two easily read -- GRACE and PEACE. The other one, HOPE, was in a little more difficult to read place, in the room but not in my line of sight. I changed that today. HOPE is in my line of site. GRACE and PEACE are deep down in me, maybe in the Lutheran part (Hah!). I am such a visual learner, though, that I wanted HOPE right there where I can see it. Done. This is a good way to start the year.

So, with HOPE in sight, these are a few of my "thankful-ness-es"

1) "a good start" at putting decorations away (to be done before chemo starts Tuesday)

2) a clean kitchen

3) the one-zillion people who are currently reaching out through prayers (OK, not a zillion, it just feels like it!)

4) two daughters who do laundry

5) a warm house on this cold, blustery night

6) feeling better (yesterday I actually went to Office Max and HyVee....then I limped for 24 hours....but I did it!)

7) clean clear water to drink, even though I am having difficulty getting to that 1 gallon a day goal. Sigh.

Keep praying!
Posted Jan 3, 2012 8:25 a.m.

As we say in our family..."You're doing a good job, and you look good doing it!" Thanks all mat-carriers...
Headed for chemo....

No Chemo After All
Posted Jan 3, 2012 2:33 p.m.

No chemo for me this week. The liver is better, but not "better enough." The same with my white count. Even my port was acting a little funny (not "hah hah" funny, though), so they had to get blood from my arm.

So, one more week to wait. At least now I know that it has been hard for me to drink all this water because my liver is swollen a bit, hence the discomfort. Dr. Mo assures me that this does not mess up the study or my participation in it. Now he knows how my body responds to this chemo, and how to protect it even better next time.

Holding....
Posted Jan 5, 2012 1:04 a.m.

About supper time, a friend invited me to go for pie at Village Inn tonight as some of our friends gather after choir at their respective places of worship. Oh, yes, and the pie is free. I was surrounded by friendship throughout the evening. These are some of the people who hold me in prayer every day. That is a good way to be held.

After I came home this evening I remembered Dr. Mo saying that my life does not need to be on hold, just because my chemotherapy session is.

Tomorrow, Sarah and I are going to see a movie. Friday I will get a hair cut. And the next day there will be something else.

All possible, because I am held in prayer, and held in the gracious grasp of God's grace. (...and in some strange trance of alliteration....)

Things that help, Part 7
Posted Jan 7, 2012 12:12 a.m.

Simple stuff....
1) Water, which is getting easier to drink more of each day.
2) Laughter with friends.
3) The satisfaction of cleaning out a closet.
4) Baking a German Chocolate cake, a family favorite.

5) The fun of black squirrel and song bird competition at the bird feeders.
6) Sunny, warm winter days.
7) Camels, laden with wise people and gifts, finally making it to worship the Child of God....the sweet satisfaction of being in the right place at the right time under the brightest star at long last. Happy Epiphany to one and all.

Second Chemo; "take two"
Posted Jan 9, 2012 8:50 p.m.

Well, I have done all that I can do to get myself ready for my second-run at my second chemo session....the food, the prayer, the meds, the prayer, the rest, the prayer, the water consumption, the prayer. My new yellow robe (made by my mom for me for Christmas) has been washed and carefully folded and is in my backpack along with everything else that I can pack the night before. I have an amazing Brookstone backpack. It is now my "go to" luggage for chemo. It keeps the laptop safe. The clothing, slippers, robe, Bible, meds, books, my favorite yellow/white LIVEstrong socks, power cords, camel, Suduko book, Action Figure Jesus with posable arms and gliding action, toothbrush, snacks and such are all ready. However, it is more than "stuff" that I have packed. I also take my nursing knowledge, my sense of humor, my family (always with me even if they aren't in the room), my mat carriers, my faith. I would say I take Jesus, but that's not true, for God truly takes me. If this were all up to me there is just no way I could do it. I feel a bit like a freshman girl ready to ask my second upperclassman to a Sadie Hawkins Dance, having been turned down on the first try. It takes some courage to put myself back out there. But, do this I will and I ask God (who is taking me) to help and guide me.

Hurray! Chemo #2 is here!
Posted Jan 10, 2012 4:16 p.m.

It took almost 6 hours to get going, but as of 2:45 p.m., the second round of chemo is running! At 2:45 p.m. tomorrow, it should be done. Dr. Mo says my labs have all recovered well. He has pulled out some super-powerful-anti-nausea-antacid-liver-protecting "trifecta" of pre-meds which took almost two hours to get going.
Now for a bit of a nap, after some more water, of course.

Complaining...
Posted Jan 11, 2012 12:39 p.m.

This morning, with my headache and exhaustion and lack of motivation to do anything besides sit in my yellow robe under the covers, I complain. Oh bother. My mind goes back to the Israelites having been freed from slavery and then complaining about the food or lack of it. They wondered why they couldn't they just go back to slavery, and food? (Exodus 16) What did they get to eat? "Manna" (which literally means "what is this?") and quail for 40 years. How did they do this? I find myself bored and frustrated with cheerios and apples and no more diet pop, no occasional glass of wine, or coffee, caffeinated tea, lots of chocolate, spicy food, or whatever else doesn't sound good at the moment. However, the Exodus story isn't about the whining complainers, it is about God's faithfulness for the full length of time that the people are in need. That brings me hope today. What I have to do mostly isn't my idea, but God will fulfill with what I need -- "my manna" -- at just the right time and place. That is where my complaining meets divine Hope. This Hope does not disappoint.

Still in Iowa, and a request
Posted Jan 11, 2012 5:02 p.m.

This chemo trip has given me bonus hours to the original 24 hours. Everything took a long time to start. Now Dr. Mo has ordered extra IV fluids. Everyone one wants me to do better on the chemo this time.

My research nurse has these thoughts; "Tell that great support group you have to even redouble their prayers on these days. They are awesome and they love you. AND think about ways to decrease stress and increase humor in your life....funny movies....fun with friends. Of course she is telling me this while I am just bawling.

The new meds, great nurses, Sarah and Erica's help -- all supportive. Lord, please let it be better this time around. Amen.

I hate it when...
Posted Jan 13, 2012 12:35 a.m.

I hate it when I figure out how to use the Netflix on the Wii....and the nausea gets about four steps ahead of me. This hasn't been a good day. Dr. Mo directed me to some meds that have helped, which is good, as I have no desire to visit the local emergency room for IV fluids and meds. The seas are stormy; please pray for "righting this ship."

Keep praying...new address
Posted Jan 13, 2012 8:10 p.m.

Well....I've made my way back to Iowa city.....I've lost my ability to spell....I've tossed 24 hours worth of cookies. I'm not at the end of my rope, but can count the fibers from this distance....Bleh, I hate nausea.

So...we'll see what they can do for me here. Keep praying....it can help us both.

A visitor
Posted Jan 14, 2012 2:39 p.m.

Cast all your anxiety on him because he cares for you. 1 Peter 5:7
Repeat as needed.

Dr. Mo came in to see me today. That helped me. And, he's used to hearing me cry anyway.

Here is his school of chemotherapy: 70% of people with chemo have no problems with side effects; 30% have a problem. Two-thirds of these problems can be severe, but get better over days. The remaining 10% have such troubles that the doctor and patient have to ask the questions "Is it worth it in terms of benefit? Is it harmful and without any good effects?" Sometimes the people in that 10% group have amazing results -- and that answers the question about proceeding, even though the chemo is crappy. For others, without measurable and effective results, it is time to move on to another treatment.

Dr. Mo figures I am probably in that 10% group. My liver is recovering because it has gotten a smaller dose of the chemo this time. I trust him. We will figure this out. He says I will need to be in the hospital until I am getting better....better stomach, liver, and fewer aches.

It is hard to limit visits to only my daughters and parents, and say no to visits from other friends. I just feel so lousy.

When Dr. Mo's nurse said they received a huge bag of treats for Dr. Mo and his staff, because he is treating "Pastor Laura." I couldn't figure out who did that, but thank you. It may not be "you" who visits, but the Holy Spirit brings your love and care right here and I am thankful.

The case for memory
Posted Jan 16, 2012 11:48 a.m.

This morning, I am reminded of why memory was a big part of my medicine. A lot of yesterday was the pits, and memory helped.
Erica and Sarah know that I love stories, so they told me my favorites.
I remembered Rodney and how very hard he strived to heal for the girls and me, and I drew on his courage. I also miss him with my whole heart. It is a blessing to remember him and see him in the quirks and joys and stories and talent and fun of our family.
 And it is good to remember that when I had my first round of chemo, I did get to feeling better after a few weeks. It is so good to know that this will get better.

"set back..."
Posted Jan 16, 2012 11:25 p.m.

I am warmed by prayers and stories today....better through the morning and early afternoon and then 'set back' by intestines that want to go on strike. Oh bother.
I sure sure do want to go home tomorrow.

Home...headed there this afternoon
Posted Jan 17, 2012 2:03 p.m.

Right now the miracle of mom's home made chicken 'n wild rice soup is buoying me for the trip. Let's do this...

Something to do immediately
Posted Jan 18, 2012 11:00 a.m.

One lovely luxury of being home again is waking and eating when I need to on my own body's timetable. Of late, it is about every two hours that I need something small to eat. That is my "immediately thing"....eating. It is a part of the second week of chemo workin' on me. I'm learning a lot about dyspepsia (basically post-chemo indigestion).

Today, in my re-introduced "time in the recliner," drinking my water, letting the meds get to working, and Bible study time, I am back into reading the lectionary. We are in the year of Mark's Gospel. I love how he gets right down to to stuff. *"Euthus"* -- roughly translated from the Greek as "immediately." In the reading for this coming Sunday (Mark 1:14-29) Jesus calls Simon, Andrew, James and John from their nets as fishermen to *immediately* come work for Jesus.

I am an "immediately" person too -- except when I procrastinate. I find it very frustrating to have to focus on the immediacy of my physical health management -- *especially* when it seems to go backwards or sideways instead of forward.

I hear of people from my church who are struggling and I want to be well and walking with them in person -- not still in the recliner at 9:35 a.m.

Maybe that is because I feel brave and faithful and courageous when I care for others. When it is me and my body I sit in worry and lack patience. I wonder when, if ever, I will feel better. I have to take little steps all the time, trusting that the big steps will come only when the little ones are all strung together. My hospital chaplain suggests that after so many years of focus on strength and courage, it is incredibly important for me to be OK with my weaknesses, and in my weakness, to rely on Christ's strength. The "doing" of this journey seems so very much bigger than I can comprehend.

So, what is helping? I'm going to name a few things....maybe they can help you cope too....or at least not feel so alone.

1) Telling me stories....especially funny ones from some trip or activity we had done together...or what we survived in raising our kids or taking classes together.

2) Sharing word/strains of hymn/songs stick in my head in beautiful ways.

3) For those who know my daughters well....checking in on them.

4) Helping me look forward to little things to do ahead....cookie baking or watching a movie or playing cards.

5) Knowing that my not contacting you isn't because I don't care, it is because I am having to do something immediately for myself....even if that is just sitting quietly in a chair waiting for meds to take effect.

86

6) Reminding me of how far I have come since the hip surgery. Chemo is different, but that surgery was still hard.

7) Just saying "Hey!" or "Still praying" speaks/prays yourself present in my and my family's life.

Things that help, Part 8
Posted Jan 19, 2012 12:22 p.m.

Yesterday I confessed weakness, worry, hopelessness, fear, and impatience. To be my "best me," I had been feeling like I needed to be strong, courageous, and patient.

So, what did I offer God? My brokenness. That's what I had. The Chaplain at U of I Hospital, helped me realize that I was letting some little pastoral pedestal that I had put myself on keep me from being ok with just being human.

Then, yesterday, without much of a fanfare at all, blessing after blessing came down. I'm picturing one of those snow falls where it quietly just keeps coming down in big flakes ---covering everything in beautiful white. Every one of these blessings were visible only because I had first offered up my weakness. My only strength is God's strength. I wish this hadn't been so hard to figure out.

A full day ahead....
Posted Jan 22, 2012 7:04 p.m.

It is a big big day tomorrow with many appointments, scans, and labs. My Australian friend (via years at Wartburg Seminary) Tanya Witwer is added to my crew for the day. I feel good about God's love and have hope for these next steps on the journey. Oh what a difference it makes to have my stomach feel better.

Tanya and I "looked ahead" in Mark 1 to the healing of Simon Peter's mother-in-law in Capernaum. I've been there, in the church built over that historical site. It is just a few yards from the synagogue in that town. While I felt the nearness of Jesus while I was there, I feel Jesus' footprints all around me here -- walking room to room with me, encouraging me to rest, to drink more water, to breathe, to inhale the peace that the Spirit has to give as a gift.

So far, so good!
Posted Jan 23, 2012 5:13 p.m.

It was so good to see a simple table set in the *last* waiting room after the *last* test with a cup of hot chicken and wild rice soup. And, it was so good to see the hip MRI shows good healing and NO new growth of tumors of any kind. The lab tests and the lung CT will be read this week. For now, I'll just breathe.

Wrapped up....resting....warm...
Posted Jan 24, 2012 10:26 p.m.

So, I wait, as I have waited so many times before. Waiting another day or two for answers to the questions of "this window of time." So, what is working? I can tell that the chemo is making a difference in my body...my skin, nails, mouth, sense of tastes and how I digest high fiber foods have all changed.
I think that tonight is a good night to turn in early. It is a good night to go back to Philippians 4: 9 *Keep on doing the things that you have learned and received and heard and seen in me, and the God of peace will be with you.*

Still in waiting...
Posted Jan 25, 2012 4:53 p.m.

The email came, from my nurse, acknowledging that today was the day that Dr. Mo would be getting back with me. Then this, "Dr. Mo wants you to come over Thursday or Friday for a meeting to come up with a master plan for your care?" And "When would you like to come over?" Sigh.

Good News...
Posted Jan 27, 2012 2:33 p.m.

Today, my family and I had the great privilege of hearing another kind of Good News. After two rounds of experimental Trabectedin chemotherapy, my lung tumors have officially *stopped growing*. (I added "officially" because I think it sounds great.) They are still there, but not bigger.

The longer part of the meeting with Dr. Mo was spent on what I want to do next. He pointed out that I have had and will continue to have a lousy physical reaction to this chemotherapy. He has and will continue to use all meds at his disposal to help with that, but that more chemotherapy of this med will/would likely be just as lousy. I'm in the "10%" of folks that this happens to. So, he laid out some options for me:

1) Keep on the chemo with a slight dose reduction, knowing I will feel pretty bad and could need hospitalization after the chemo like I did this last time.
2) Stop the chemo.....stop the study.....go on an eight week break from chemo then re-test....if it is growing again, start a different chemo (as this experimental drug that works on it will no longer be available to me).
3) Rest for the next week....let my liver labs come back in line and my white count come back in line....wait/think/pray about what I want to do next.
The big thing that he impressed upon all of us was that I did not *have* to do anything, ever, or right now even. The choice to do chemotherapy is mine alone.
Right now, I am choosing #3.....rejoicing that my tumors have stopped growing, and resting. This is good work to do. I wish that I could say I felt good all the time, but I don't. That liver inflammation is no fun. The effects of chemo on my skin, nails, teeth, and gums, is kicking in too. However, right now, my cancer is at a *full stop* and I am absolutely *fully* thankful.

The kitchen drawer, a poke in the eye, and a strategy.

Posted Jan 31, 2012 10:50 a.m.

A couple of years ago I remodeled the kitchen. We love it. It is a small kitchen that works. Of course, it's not "self-cleaning." I couldn't afford that in the budget. One drawer in particular seems to be the most in disarray all the time....the one with the twist-ties, candle lighters, screwdrivers, and dried out Sharpies.

With that image in mind, I take you back to last Friday and Saturday. It was as if I invited all 650-plus of you into my "newly remodeled kitchen" and *everyone* was thrilled with it -- couldn't be happier! Only the "Newly Remodeled Kitchen" was my lungs, where the tumors had *stopped* growing. This was and is amazing news. The thing is, as much as I wanted to, I couldn't party with you. I was stuck, picking through that one drawer full of odds and ends...stuff I found but not when I needed it. Really, a junk drawer. I truly did want that remodeled kitchen (new and improved lungs) *and* I wanted more. I wanted all the junk that goes with that healing to just go away. It is hard to explain the "drawer" when the "room" looks so amazing. And, there I was stuck for about 3 1/2 days, mainly crying, with a side of despair.

The origin of the despair?
1) I still felt pretty horrible. I had already had a border-line migraine-level headache for 4-5 days and couldn't figure out why. I still have some sort of nausea a few times a day if my eating gets messed up. And, I have some sort of liver pain 30% of the day or more.
2) I was grieving. My "plan" reads like this: Laura has chemo. Laura has very few side effects from chemo. Laura's chemo works. Laura can get back to some level of work as her treatment continues. This is not what I got.
3) I was given choices by Dr. Mo. I elected wait/pray/think. For some reason I felt like I was trying to win a no-win scenario. Only, I couldn't win it. I kept coming back to Dr. Mo explaining that I would get sick

90

every time I had that chemo. Folks, it is hard to poke yourself in the eye with a stick, when there is still a stick in there from the first time you did it.

So here I am, overcome with apprehension, fear, worry, anxiety, related to *everything* about chemotherapy. The thought of being sick to my stomach made me sick to my stomach! Memories from the hospital of late food, cold food, and strong medications colored everything. In the midst of it all I found myself powerless to change those thoughts.

And, you all were happy for me. I so wanted to be happy for myself. And yet my doctor admitted that it could all happen again, every time. I don't know what your demons look like. But that is certainly mine. The thought came to me that this is Post Traumatic Stress Syndrome. And I cried some more, and waited for the call from my counselor on Monday afternoon.

Over the course of the hour long call, with my counselor's help, I reoriented myself to what was truly real. I learned to ask the questions: Am I in danger now? Am I safe now? Am I throwing up now? No. Yes. No. Then he helped me develop strategies for the situations I could be in with chemo. For instance, I will take my own food to the hospital. I will have someone stay with me at the hospital again for chemo, *and* I will have someone stay with me overnight if I have to go back in (I sent people home before).

So, in the grand scheme, I would have had chemo today. However, given what my liver labs were on Friday, I don't think I would have "passed the test" and been allowed to begin. I look forward to feeling better this week. I look forward to being happy *with* you all about the *NO GROWTH OF TUMORS*.

How good? ... "Free pie" good
Posted Feb 2, 2012 10:24 a.m.

For the first time in literally months, I feel good. The capstone of February 1 was a trip to Village Inn at 8:15 p.m. for a time of laughter with friends and pie. Wednesday = FREE pie. My favorite pie is Triple Berry.

For me, that pie is all grace (grace = undeserved, unearned love). Granted, for some it might seem a stretch or even a leap to go from free pie at Village Inn to God's grace (a gift beyond ALL measure), but certainly that pie "reminds" me of God's grace, most especially now, because God's grace is meant to be lived out in *community*. In Jesus' time many illnesses kept people from being in community. Certainly cancer can still have that effect. So for me, to eat that free pie *and* to eat it in the community of friends is one gift on top of another. (Triple Berry Pie enjoyment is also made possible by my sponsors -- Prilosec and Prevacid.)

Because I know that by next Wednesday evening I won't be feeling "free-pie-good," I will enjoy it now...offer thanks for it now...and look forward to feeling this good again, even if it takes a month.

This side of the mat...
Posted Feb 3, 2012 12:02 p.m.

Today I have a precious image in my mind: you all carrying me on the mat to see Jesus.

A few days ago, a friend asked if I had ever had a friend who was seriously ill. I said yes, and related what that was like...frustrations, feelings of helplessness, wishing there was something I could do besides pray, feelings of grief, wondering if I could/should call especially if I hadn't in a while. "From this side of the mat," I say to never underestimate the power of your prayers, and the power of making contact. I keep trying to look for redemptive parts of this illness, and if it brings friends back together in new ways, that is a blessing.

Thinking "opposite" with food
Posted Feb 4, 2012 8:15 p.m.

Many years ago, after Rod's death from colon cancer, I started telling every one over fifty to get a colonoscopy. Even through Rod died at forty-six, fifty is the "usual" age that insurance companies start paying for that procedure. Around that time I also started to increase the fiber in my diet, just for good colon health in general.

However, now, as my next chemotherapy approaches, I know that I need to do something different! Today, I thank my sweet cousin Sheryl (Davis) Svoboda, dietician with cancer patients at Loyola, for helping me think through what I need to do to tolerate the effects of my treatment and still have food taste good! The chemotherapy shuts down my gastro-intestinal system. Therefore, I need food that is more easily digestible. This calls for low fiber, and minimal meat protein in the early days. I have to admit I will miss my whole grain bread and oatmeal and apples, but white bread, cream of wheat, and applesauce are calling my name now. I know that after week three, I can go back to eating some of the stuff I love.

Hopefully tomorrow I will feel well enough for worship because there is a meal there of bread and wine that I love more than *any* other meal I have, any other day of the week.

A gift....
Posted Feb 7, 2012 10:17 p.m.

There are all sorts of things that can be considered gifts....gifts of the Spirit....birthday gifts and such. I guess it could be said that I sewed that Valentine skirt for Erica as a "gift," however I think I was the one who got the greater gift. Having that project to do before this chemo session gave me something to focus on. I also remember seeing the pattern and the slippery fabric and thinking at first, how difficult the skirt would be to fit and make. Then, I thought, "You know what? You have cancer. THAT is something hard to fix. This skirt is nothin'...in fact, it is a JOY in comparison." I guess it is the gift of perspective. It is also something that people have helped me with --- cutting out the pattern, phone-coaching, cheering me on.... and now that skirt is done! And, Erica loves it. I find that my chemo sessions are much the same as making that skirt, with many people involved in helping me prepare and "live through" and heal through the experience. Everybody's help is a gift.

No chemo today for me...
Posted Feb 8, 2012 4:30 p.m.

Everything went so very smoothly this morning -- packing the cooler, the bags, the vehicle, the drive, the arrival on the unit, the "port access," the blood drawing, the EKG....and then the waiting for the results of the blood test. So here is the deal: my liver has a "grade 2" problem. If it was a "grade 1" problem like four other lab results are, it would be no problem, but grade 2 is a problem. It means "no chemo for me" this week. It means coming back home, doing what I do, drinking plenty of water, eating good food, resting, enjoying life....and then going back on Valentine's Day to try again.

A little help here...
Posted Feb 11, 2012 12:21 a.m.

I eat good foods. I drink plenty of water.
However, I am letting my mind fuss over whether or not I'll be having chemo next week. This is odd as a few weeks ago I wasn't sure I wanted it ever again. I can still stay in the clinical trial, even if I have to wait another week. Still, I seem to be worrying over this like a tongue over a chip in a tooth. Worry is a natural place to see on the journey, but it is not my intended destination. So, I guess that is where I ask for your prayers.

Already the best Valentine...
Posted Feb 13, 2012 8:06 p.m.

In Owego School, my elementary school in rural Livingston County, Illinois, Valentine's Day was a much loved and long anticipated day. Certainly there was a party at school. I really don't remember too much about the party, except for two things: that we exchanged Valentines with our classmates, AND that the Valentines were delivered into each person's Valentine Box. I LOVED making Valentine boxes. The older I got, the more complicated (and totally lovely) the box would be. I don't remember ever seeing a picture around of these boxes, but I remember one year my box had a "ramp" for the cards to slide down. (Perhaps the fact that the incline was too flat and the cards didn't exactly roll down the ramp, would offer evidence for why I passed on engineering as a career choice.)

This year I didn't make a box, and the day hasn't even arrived, but it is already one of my favorite Valentine "years." Why? Because of the time I got to spend with my daughters -- making Valentine cards with Sarah at the dining room table and preparing for Erica's Valentine's party with her. These are simple things, but so appreciated.

Yesterday in worship, I heard the story of the healing of Naaman from his leprosy (2 Kings 5). He was told to do the simplest thing -- go wash seven times in the Jordan. Eventually he did and was healed. He had resisted doing this simple thing. Shouldn't healing take some fancy effort? As I heard the Word...I remembered the simple thing I have been told to do -- drink water. That's all. This last week I have really been "pouring it in!" And, I have noticed that it has been easier, actually. This simple thing is a gift I am giving myself.

The other gift I gave myself, was the gift of asking for help. I told God and you all about my worrying, and it has been much relieved in these last days. In fact, the more I asked for help, the more I was blessed with support from every corner. Those are gifts of love...

Hurray for a "good liver!"
Posted Feb 14, 2012 4:57 p.m.

The Cancer Center waiting room was the third one we had waited in this morning, but the first with good news -- my liver is healed enough to begin chemotherapy! I talked with Dr. Mo privately a bit later. He said that the "good" that I feel now at five weeks away from chemotherapy is because the cancer has been *stopped*. Really? Really.

Breathing
Posted Feb 18, 2012 11:41 p.m.

is helped by
1) having loving people around me to help me keep focused.
2) having those same people feed me good food.
3) having insurance to pay for medicines that work.
4) having that truck that parked on me yesterday, move over today.
5) some time with my daughters.
6) friends who check in through the day.
7) keeping it all in perspective.
8) the gift of hope.
9) the Breath of Life.
10) not having to be in the hospital this time around for chemo follow up. This is big.

Near and Far
Posted Feb 21, 2012 12:30 a.m.

About a half hour ago Mom and I got home from the Emergency Room at Trinity-Rock Island. It was snowing big white flakes that had covered everything in the hour that we were there. I really appreciate the care that I get in Iowa City and I'm so very glad that that hospital and care givers are there. However, I'm also glad to have good hospitals right in town.
When I was in the hospital for chemo last week one of my IV sites in my right arm "quit working." The site has continued to hurt...and had started swelling a bit and was getting warmer than the rest of my arm. I talked with Dr. Mo via email and followed his advice to get it checked out.
Now, I'm home, on antibiotics and so sleepy. As I left the hospital, I saw a friend whose loved one is in the hospital. I don't look too much like myself at 11 p.m. with no make up, so I said who I was, and we talked briefly. It seemed we both needed to know that God is not only in far away medical

centers. I'm not glad I had to go get checked out at the hospital, but I am glad to be where a friend needed to hear the same thing that I did. God is here.

Remember...
Posted Feb 22, 2012 10:46 a.m.

"Remember that you are dust, and to dust you shall return." For eight years (plus seminary internship) these were words I shared -- proclaimed -- whispered -- as I made the sign of the cross in ashes on people's foreheads on Ash Wednesday. Doing so was a lot like preaching because I couldn't say "It's so" for someone else and not accept it for myself as well. This Ash Wednesday is different from any other I have experienced. I'll be asking a friend to bring me ashes rather than receive them in worship. It makes me realize once again the importance of the Body of Christ, especially when separated from that Body as it worships regularly. I guess the kicker for me this time is that almost every day since late September I have considered my "dust-i-ness" (mortality). This way of being is the short-term-on-earth-sort-of-getting-around. And, based on my actions toward keeping my "dust" in the best-possible-health, it appears that I am pretty much all for staying on this side of the "dust line"…six feet over, instead of six feet under. What an odd place to be....fully looking at my "dust-i-ness" in the face, and fully confident in God's amazing plans for the resurrection, and every day taking full steps to make sure that the only part of me that goes to the dust right now are tumors.

Have you ever seen one of those really intricate "sand pictures"? Not the pictures one might make with the side of your hand, just pushing piles of sand around. No, I mean the ones where it looks like a huge amazing rug or design on the floor -- I think the images are made as a part of a religious practice, but I can't remember the faith tradition. They are remarkable. And when they are done, they are swept up. The images are left to their memories and the iPhones of the tourists.

I admit that I have a much better appreciation of that dust/sand when it is in a beautiful design than when it is swept up and recycled to whereever

97

dust/sand goes. However, I don't think that is how God operates. When I remember that I am dust, I also remember that God loves this dust (and all y'all's dust)...when it is all new and fresh and in order, and when it is out of order and broken, too. And (CPR and all resuscitation skills aside), it is God who breathes life into dust, not us. (Given my mom's cleaning efforts on my behalf this week, it would seem that I might have some sort of an advanced degree in dust collection, however...)

Perhaps, this Ash Wednesday more than any other, I give thanks that God "breathes life" into this dust.

Giving myself...
Posted Feb 24, 2012 8:54 p.m.

OK....I admit that my attitude toward "being my best me" in my lifetime has quite often meant going way above and beyond what I really needed to do. Many people have called me "driven" -- sometimes even to my face! So, it shouldn't be any surprise to me that when I started really truly feeling better late yesterday and early today that I wanted to be "better faster!" I wanted to know why I was feeling better -- so I could keep doing whatever that was! Right?! Not so much. It is stressful not to leave (in this case) "well enough, alone." My Lenten discipline today has been to "give myself a break," to feel better, and not stress about being better than the better I already am.

A few "visits" ago with Dr. Mo, I was feeling pretty well and I told him so. He said, "Isn't that great?! That is what it feels like when the cancer isn't growing." What a good feeling that is. I am trying to keep telling myself that very thing. I am also not pushing myself to stop taking medicine for pain. I tried that recently and realized quickly that walking was more difficult, and that I ached all over. Yep. There it is. So, I'm giving myself a break, being my best me, and feeling better with pain meds -- better enough for today.

Maybe this can help me live out what Paul said to the Corinthians (2 Cor. 12:9)..... *But he said to me, "My grace is sufficient for you, for my power is made perfect in weakness." Therefore I will boast all the more gladly about my weaknesses, so that Christ's power may rest on me."*

Still giving...
Posted Feb 25, 2012 11:27 a.m.

Yesterday, I got an email with an attached picture from Dee, Rod's sister. The picture was one of Rod's grave, next to their dad Ervin's grave, with a new bouquet of flowers in the vase. Over these last seven plus years, as a family, we have kept flowers on Rod's grave. It is a tricky thing for me to accomplish because I live over two hours away. I appreciated seeing the picture in addition to the action because today is Rod's birthday. He would have been 54. I can't say that his birthday is an "easy" day, but certainly in the years since his death our minds are more filled with funny and loving stories than the stories that broke our hearts from his illness.

Today I am celebrating Rod's life by giving thanks for the ways he gave to us.... the gift of our two daughters, the sense of humor, the "move with his wife yet again" as she gets another graduate degree, the support of my pastoring, the gift of music, and the gift of his faith. He is still giving.

Given a baby to hold...
Posted Feb 27, 2012 1:02 p.m.

Maybe today gave me a bit of a new perspective on Jesus welcoming the children (Mark 10:13-16). Jesus' sidekicks were none too happy that Jesus would want to see the hoards of children that parents kept bringing to him that day. Honestly, how could Jesus be a mover and a shaker if he decided to hang out with these children who had nothing to offer? Right? I preferred to hear the story from the perspective of the parents of those kids -- parents who were so thankful and hopeful to get their children in the hands of someone who loved them all...and could bring healing too, if that was needed. Jesus even told them that the reign of God was like this -- with Jesus in the center and children of God surrounding him -- love obviously going both ways.

This morning, at the same time as a visit from the Total Maintenance repair guy, I got a visit from a new mommy and daddy, colleagues of mine, and their eight-week-old daughter. They asked if I would like to hold her. I said yes, of course, and that I had washed my hands already!

For the next ten minutes you could not convince me that there was a care in the whole wide world. Of the four of us, I'm not sure who smiled more. Honestly, that is some good and powerful medicine. I absolutely love babies. This one was no exception. A gift of joy, dressed in pink. As I was given the opportunity to hold this sweet child, I was also given the chance to be reminded of how God loves all God's children....me and mine....you and yours....even when we think we are being a bother to an otherwise busy Savior....there is always time for a visit....Jesus just loves it.

Given another chance
Posted Feb 28, 2012 2:18 p.m.

The Oscars provided a time for me to make some progress on my first knitting project -- a washcloth with a butterfly pattern on it. At row thirteen, I found too many stitches. I took out two rows to get out of the patterned area and called mom to make sure I knew how to reduce the stitches and get back on target. That project will resume tonight. I needed a break from it...it was a little disheartening to count up to 37 instead of 35 over and over as I checked and rechecked. Where did those unwanted stitches come from. I know I only had 35 to start with!

Last night as I did my devotions and then read for a bit, I thought about the "extra stuff" I had and have in me. I thought about what has been taken out and what has been bathed in chemotherapy -- and stopped from growing. I remembered that God has known me from my first knitting...as I was being formed.

Those two unwanted stitches gave me something...they gave me another chance to be thankful for the many people who have helped me go from "37 to 35" so-to-speak. My physical healing is certainly more complicated than this butterfly-patterned-peach-colored washcloth.....but both are exercises in patience.

Given a mixed bag
Posted Feb 29, 2012 6:50 p.m.

Today seemed sort of a mixed bag for me. I spent a good portion of the day checking my email to see if my lab results were in. The longer I waited, the more I focused on the what-if situations that could occur. Then a phone call came from a friend. A mutual friend and colleague had died after a long fight with cancer. My heart breaks for the spouse, children and extended family.

The U.S. news has been filled with pictures of communities suffering because they were in the path of rare February tornados. Many lost their lives as well as their homes. Then, the image of one of my first "star-crushes" -- Davy Jones -- who recently died of a heart attack.

In the middle of these life changing events for so many, a friend came by with a treat and prayer, a package and some cards came, and the labs came back -- the best ever at two weeks after chemo with only one liver enzyme at Grade 1 lousy.

Having lived through some of those days where it seemed all bad, I found myself especially thankful for the lovely things of this day. Then I found myself feeling bad because I had had a good day, when so many had such difficult days.

I remembered how people expressed some of those same things to me when Rod died, and when I was diagnosed. I remembered saying this: "It's not a contest." It is going to happen that a terrible day for one is a great (or at least okay) day for another.

The thing that is the same in these situations is that Christ is present in all of them...in joy and in sorrow, present in this life, and welcoming my friend into the next.

Given a gift from the earth
Posted Mar 1, 2012 9:35 p.m.

Years ago, after Rod died, I was home with the girls for a month before returning to ministry. I really don't remember much from those days. However, one thing I do remember was the day that two friends came over to the house, dressed warmly (it was November) and took me outside. They showed me dozens of bulbs that they brought for the three of us to plant. An hour later we had planted bulbs, and hope, just a little hope, that some day wouldn't be so gray or so cold, and there would be new life again.
Just as they said, a few months later, the crocuses and then a few weeks later some beautiful tulips showed up and so did hope, and the reminder that after death comes new life.
Today wasn't my best day. It wasn't my worst day (by any means). Rather, it was day with moments where the events of the last five months loomed large. It was the right day to walk out side, feel the sunshine, and take a picture of a bit of nature's beauty that showed up again. (With a picture it is easier to remember.) Sometimes reminders of the good news are only a few inches tall...and lavender.

Given one stitch at a time
Posted Mar 2, 2012 11:40 p.m.

Yesterday was a good day to take outdoor pictures, like pictures of crocuses, and pictures of knitting (this could be a surprise as knitting isn't typically an "outdoor sport).. Today, those same locations are covered in over two inches of slushy snow. Good thing I brought the knitting back inside. ☺
Today I started actively preparing for next Tuesday's chemo session. I haven't wanted to think so much about it beyond. Yes. Let's do this.

I'll be ready with a parallel pep talk for my liver. However, today I started making my lists of things to take or to remember to do ahead. It helped to talk to Penny and to Erica about this. It turns out that after a few hours into the treatment I don't remember everything about the experience. Fortunately, the friends and family that have been a part of my chemo and lab experiences are very understanding of this, and/or save their chuckles for another time.

My butterfly patterned wash cloth knitting project is half way done. I feel a bit like that wash cloth....not all there, but I've got a message of new life (resurrection) and I'm getting there one stitch at a time.

Given another day to wait
Posted Mar 6, 2012 5:01 p.m.

Well, just when the liver is all "spiffy," the neutrophil count is lacking. Of course it took four hours, accessing my port twice, countless syringes and doses of heparin. Sigh....

Dr. Mo was in good spirits and very encouraging, however. I am now on steroids today and tonight and will go west again tomorrow (with all we packed up today) and try again. I did find out that this next time I will not need an extra IV site, for which I am *very* thankful! They will let me know tomorrow when my next round of scans will be.

So, y'all praying-mat-carriers, carry on, you do fine work.

Given good results
Posted Mar 7, 2012 5:07 p.m.

Well, the computer access won't work in my patient room, but I, and my mom/back scratcher, and my IV pole with chemo meds running, have found our way to a computer in the waiting room. The port was no more interested in running today than yesterday....they actually used the meds on it that they use on folks when they have strokes and do some "clot busting." It is working marginally better.

However, know this; my neutrophil count not only went up "31" from 1470 to 1501, it went up to over 3330. Yep, I'm rockin' the neutrophils.

Given a green day....
Posted Mar 12, 2012 6:29 p.m.

This is my green day. This is my day to fully live in-to my frog-i-ness (fully relying on God). The rain last night is bringing on the green in my lawn. I'm wearing a green shirt. I'm fixin' to get ready to knit a bright green frog patterned wash cloth (as I will finish my second yellow wash cloth tonight). I have plenty of frog stuff around me to remind me to rely on God....including a great book mark, two new frog pillow cases, a frog wind chime, and a frog patterned blanket all within my view from my late afternoon siesta on my bed. I smile thinking of the vast collection of frog stuff in my study at church. It seems now that for as many times as I told my fully rely on God (FROG) stories in my ministry that I was just warming myself up to tell those same stories to myself in these past months.

Tomorrow is a leap-of-faith day. I'll need all my good frog stuff on board. Tomorrow is my three-month scan day (MRI of my hip and CT of my chest/abdomen/pelvis). That must mean that it has been three months since chemo started. Tomorrow is the day that brings on what most cancer patients call "scanxiety." I can't say that I disagree. However, this time, having had good results (a.k.a. cancer not growing larger in my lungs) last time, my scanxiety is much less this time. I'm sure that I could whip myself into a bit of a frenzy but so far haven't. If anything has me concerned about tomorrow it is having to go through the prep for the scans when I am so "fresh" off of chemo. Today was my first day without significant nausea -- and that is just because Mom is making me food as fast as I need it all day long!

I can also use some prayers that my amethyst-colored-triune-shaped-power-port does its job tomorrow! On chemo day they had to blast it with the same stuff they give folks who have had strokes just to get it open and flowing well. I expect it to perform well tomorrow!

I've elected to get my results from Dr. Mo on the phone on Wednesday rather than make another trip over.

That is where I am today. Feeling a bit frog-like, I think. Anyhow, having jumped my concerns into all of your capable praying hands and hearts I can go back to knitting, or waiting until the next meal.

Given the chance...
Posted Mar 13, 2012 9:13 p.m.

Given the chance for a new day tomorrow, I will take it for sure. Oh. My. Goodness. I do not suggest doing scans at six days after chemo. So. I will not dwell on that, but lift up the help that mom gave and lift up the power port that worked wonderfully (I did speak firmly to it before we left) and lift up the great staff of the MRI and CT areas that helped me and my port through the day, and lift up all y'all for your support as well. Some day soon the aches and nausea will ease up. Some time tomorrow, Dr. Mo will call and we will breathe and take what ever step is next.

Given good news...
Posted Mar 14, 2012 7:58 p.m.

It is about 6:45 p.m. on Wednesday, March 14. ("pi" day for the 3.14 observant...). I'm still awaiting a conversation with Dr. Mo. However, around 4:15 this afternoon he reviewed my MRI and CT scans and posted the results to "mychart" (the on-line site where I can see all of my lab tests, reports, etc at University of Iowa Hospital & Clinics). After he posted them, they were available for me to see. I saw them about an hour later -- so what did he see? NO NEW GROWTH! Hurray!
I had thought that I would wait until he called to post something, but good news (similar to the Good News of Jesus) just needs to be shared....and I have no idea if Dr. Mo will call yet tonight.
So....tonight, after you are done doing stuff like dancing because of this good news, or joining me in praying our thanks, or watching American Idol, or enjoying the amazing weather.... continued prayers for these ol' chemo side effects to be so-over-with would be great. (I had such good results with the port and tumor prayers, that I have to ask!)
Growing faith, not tumors, on the journey.

Given a day to feel a little better...
Posted Mar 16, 2012 11:55 p.m.

"We want to go home....there's no food, no water...just this miserable manna...whatever that is....and now we're being killed off by snakes!" What a great story. Moses takes care of it for God, though. That bronze snake on a pole is just the thing to look at to get better quick. (Hear the full story in Numbers 21 in a Bible near you....)
Oh, my goodness. This is day nine from the start of chemo round four. It has been no where *near* 40 years and honestly I can sense my inner-Israelite coming out in me. If the major achy-ness hadn't passed, who knows what God would have been hearing.

Given some cuts...
Posted Mar 19, 2012 11:22 p.m.

So. What would be good things to do or at least try to do as I feel better? Besides knit, that is. Well, I offered to finish the t-shirt quilt that Sarah completed the top and back for. It is made of fifteen-inch squares of t-shirt fronts or backs. Seventy shirts or so are used. The front and back of the quilt is sewn together, and is laid out on the living room floor, ready to have the edges cut evenly, then the sewing-together and machine quilting will begin. I started on the "evening-out" of the edges while Sarah was home for break but didn't feel well enough to get it finished. So, yesterday, late afternoon I got back to it. FYI -- *don't* use one hand and one foot to hold a yardstick in place as you run the rotary cutter, because you might cut the top of your big toe in the process. Oh, my goodness. A big toe can bleed, for goodness sake. Now I am working quite hard to keep that wound from opening up. (applying pressure, elevating the foot...) While I didn't spend the money on a completely occulusive bandaid, my mind "willed" it to be just that tight and protective. I didn't spend the $$ at Walgreen's on one though. I can accept the "water-proof" one that was in my drawer.
However, this evening, after babying the toe all day, I could take it no more. I had to get outside. It was too too lovely to miss. Many of you

know that working at some level in my yard is one of the best ways to heal my spirit, if not my toe. So, out I went with a stool and hand shears and a lawn/leaf bag. Very slowly I trimmed two small bushes back to size. God is doing such an amazing job in the yard. It felt good to be just a little bit of a partner with the process.

So with that small project done, I moved slowly to put things away, without disturbing the "toe." As I moved to the garage to put the long shears away, I saw something in the leaves by the deck. A garter snake (actually an anaconda in my memory but I'll agree to something between a cobra and a boa constrictor). We have had snakes in the yard every year for four or more. I have even removed garter snakes (half the size of this one) from the basement. (Don't be too wowed. If it was a bird that was in the house I would have sold the place rather than take care of it.) I decided that I would rather deal with this snake, than try to get my daughters to do lawn work in the coming months, knowing that that ol' snake was still there. (This one was over two feet long and not quite as big around as my big toe).

So. I took those long blade garden shears and made the snake eligible for the local spinal rehab clinic. He/she was quite disappointed in my decision, and was no more impressed with the direct flight that I gave him/her over the fence and to the far-back yard. What a relief. Then, I walked slowly back toward the house, and, what did I see? His/her brother/sister. Same size. Same location. I almost didn't do anything. That first-snake adrenaline rush was pert-n-near spent. Then, I thought of my lungs. I am not satisfied with knowing there is stuff growing there. I want it gone. Now, snake #2 is joining #1 in applying to the spinal rehab clinic. I'll tell you I looked long and hard for #3 and the rest of the herd (or gaggle or pride or whatever a bunch of snakes are called).

As I rest in the recliner drinking my water, actually thirsty for the first time in a long time, with my foot up, I find that my "cutting" is a mixed bag. I'm very disappointed with a hasty cut to my toe. Last night I was practically in tears just because I feel like everything is so very slow in my recovery this time, and this just slowed me up more. Then, those cuts to the bushes brought back just a glimmer of hope that I can do some little bits of something I love so much. Then, those snakes -- well, it embarrasses me a bit. I had a deal with the snakes that I had found in the basement. I get the inside and they can have the outside. These two snakes did not get the benefit of that earlier agreement, unless these are the ones that I released outside two years ago. Come to think of it maybe I don't feel so bad after all.

Given a chance to do it again...
Posted Mar 20, 2012 11:24 p.m.

It has been a beautiful day here. I had the opportunity to do a few things differently today...and here is it how it came out.

-- I loved the time with Erica as I rode around with her on her errands, even making a few purchases myself. She took me by South Park Presbyterian church so I could vote.

-- I sewed one side of Sarah's t-shirt quilt and stayed clear of the rotary cutter. This quilt is going to look great!

--I looked at the yard, trees and flowers but did no trimming. My back is fine, but my right hip is "angry" about the previous day's effort of sitting on that stool to trim the bushes.

--While admiring the lawn, I looked out over the back driveway and guess what I saw. Yep. The younger brother/sister of yesterday's snake twins. If I thought it would have been "catch-able" I would have called the local retired high school environmental sciences teacher to relocate "my snake" to her lovely yard habitat (per her request). Regardless, the snake lives for another day. Little does that snake know how much greener that other yard really is.

--Unfortunately, the last four hours have been pretty achy. And, for a while I wondered if I was even getting a fever. I changed my toe-dressing yet again and it looks to be healing quite well. My port is fine. I have no runny nose or cough. My temperature never got over 99 degrees, so there was no need to call Dr. Mo. Perhaps my body is just saying something about "balance." Likely that is the case. Tomorrow, I'll hang around the house and I will drink lots of water. I have to admit that it is scary to feel like the balance of my well-being is so very delicate.

Given a minute

Posted Mar 23, 2012 10:03 p.m.

Here are a couple of "minute" snapshots from today....

-Welcoming Erica home at about 3 a.m. from the midnight showing of "The Hunger Games"

-Saying good morning and good bye to Erica as she left for work at 7:30 a.m.

-and after work would travel to Dubuque to see her best friend and see "The Hunger Games" (again)

-Texting words of comfort to Sarah and praying for two families and the Illinois State University campus as they grieve the death of two students last night (one in Sarah's dorm and one in the sister dorm of hers).

-Quilting the t-shirt quilt (MANY minutes, actually)

-Watching an amazing documentary on origami on Netflix

-Watching the movie "My Left Foot" on Netflix

-Doing a crop survey of the beautiful things growing in my yard

-Eating too many cookies but not getting sick from them

-Going to my dear friend's work place to help her celebrate her birthday

-Playing the piano

-Praying for my kids

-Praying for people who are grieving

-Wondering what to take to eat for chemo next Tuesday

-Praying thanksgiving for a day with pain only in that ol' liver....

thanks be to God

Given a small sign
Posted Mar 25, 2012 12:34 a.m.

Almost two years ago now, when I returned from my travels to Israel and Germany, a dear friend set up an "oasis" of sorts on my back deck. It had sand and camels (my Fisher Price ones) and lots of fun stuff, including "signs." These signs were small post-it notes with bits of wisdom written on each with a Sharpie. I kept the signs and pulled one out today. What does it read?

"Be here now."

Sometimes it is a reminder for me to just be present. To live intentionally. Sometimes it is a prayer. "Whew! Hey Lord! Be here now! This is a mess! Help!"

This time in my chemo cycle, as I approach the Sunday and Monday before chemo, is an especially key time to practice "Be here now" as a spiritual discipline. I think it is a way of living fully in these days. At least that is what I am striving to do. During these two days, I try to have a reasonable "to do" list and have some satisfaction in completing some simple things.

To note....thinking about this, writing about this, has done precisely what the "Be here now" practice is supposed to keep me from doing. For example, I thought "Oh, yes, I need to get such and such bills paid before I go to chemo, just in case I get more ill and cannot get them paid in the first week after chemo. This got me thinking of that second chemo and being in the hospital for five extra days. And this got me a bit freaked out. I say this because I certainly don't want to set myself up as some ubber-super-focused-non-worried-cancer-person. That is just not the case. Some days the line between "handling it" and "not-handling it" is a hair's breadth.

None the less. When I say, "Be here now," I am talking both to myself and to God. We will work on this together.

Given Round #5
Posted Mar 27, 2012 2:06 p.m.

Yep, it took a few hours to find out that my fifth Chemo is a "go." My amethyst-colored-triune-shaped-Power-Port worked famously on the first try! I had a good visit with Dr. Mo about some aches and pains and the origins of said pains. While it seemed that one of my tumors may have shrunk a bit as seen in the last scan, he said that he considers it "stable disease" and then went on to describe the way they measure and what changes are considered significant. He also explained why I had such severe pain after a shopping trip with Erica around town. The additional walking (weight bearing exercise) was encouraging my bone marrow to release white blood cell production, which causes the bone and muscle pain to increase extremely. Fortunately he also increased my pain medication for those experiences. Now, I am back on track.

Given care
Posted Mar 28, 2012 11:55 p.m.

Brief tonight....poor typing skills (from chemo and meds).
I have been given the most lovely care, from my doctor and nurses, and from my family.
Fed good food in a timely way.
Head and leg rubs when I ached all over.
Stories shared.
Videos watched.
Prayers for healing.
Visit from the Lutheran UIHC chaplain, and this....especially thankful for the Lenten devotion book from Trinity Lutheran this year, with a special thanks for the devotions from the confirmands....thanks for sharing your faith....I am incredibly proud of you.

Given an update
Posted Mar 31, 2012 11:52 a.m.

This chemo round is hitting me pretty hard. At 10:30 last night, a good natured oncology fellow from UIHC talked me through some steps (over the phone) that kept me from being re-admitted. Then mom got me calmed and relaxed to try sleep. Maybe now, 12 hours later I am a half step ahead of the yuckies.

Given a window
Posted Mar 31, 2012 8:12 p.m.

In two days, I will be passing a window. The window: six months and six days. This was Rodney's window from diagnosis to death for colon cancer. Actually I feel quite confident that I will go past that window in this life. However, holding that window open for me has made me ever so tender toward the brevity of that window for him. So short. What is a good goal? His goal was forever....for his daughter's lifetimes. Certainly, for me. Can I do twelve months and twelve days? How about ten years survival? That would double down and blow past any projected "can do" rate for sarcomas which sits at around five years. Is this surviving? Sure it is. Each day is a celebration of surviving. Too bad it is so hard to do some days.

Last night after I took my anti-nausea med, I tried to meditate by breathing. I went back to that Advent practice.....sighing...and having the spirit gather my sighs and breathe back peace. But I couldn't remember the sigh part....perhaps it was more of a 'moan in pain' part. A "moan" as in I will not throw up again. I will do whatever I have to do to keep myself from being re-admitted to the hospital. Then I remembered the peace part. That I clung to. That I needed.

Given something to do
Posted Apr 2, 2012 10:49 a.m.

Today, the scripture for the Monday of Holy Week includes John 12:1-11 which has the anointing of Jesus's feet by Mary, as if he were being anointed for burial. Such an extravagance. After years of "study" on this though, I get it.

In these days the work that I am pouring myself into is managing my physical state with (1) food, (2) rest, and (3) medications (and countless other things, but these are crucial). I am missing my work as a pastor, though, and being a part of telling the story of Christ's passion in worship. I am missing the actions that come with that worship: the waving of palms, the kneeling in prayer together, the gathering of my darkest clothes to wear for Good Friday, the stripping of the altar, the meditation on scripture and preparation for preaching.

As I sit in the sun in the recliner, I am left to wonder how I might honor Christ's resurrection gift through what I can do now. How I can "be here now" with my current limitations and know that what I have to offer is truly enough? This is what I have come up with: I can

- invite people who are at my home to see everything that is blooming outside for it is a gift to the eyes and heart
- quilt a bit each day on Sarah's t-shirt quilt...bit by bit it is nearing completion
- pray for those who are also trying to strive through treatment for cancer- graciously accept the love and help of my family and friends near and far- "be here now" and to look ahead to things that bring me joy (including figuring out how to grow sunflower plants without the interference of my local bunnies and squirrels
- love and encourage my daughters
- say thank you more

Given a space to wait

Posted Apr 3, 2012 9:51 a.m.

April 3, 2012 Tuesday of Holy Week: The Gospel text is from John again (12:20-36)....after the anointing. Jesus has gone up for the festival. The Greeks want to see what Jesus is all about. Then there is all this talk about the seed that must fall to the earth and die before it rises. God talks to Jesus from heaven for the benefit of the crowd. I love to think about that time...that space...that "liminal" (threshold) space where the line between what we see and know and feel and hope that Christ is doing is all blurred.

My liminal space at home is the recliner. The recliner actually sits in the threshold between the living and dining room. It was Rod's chair. Now it's mine. Likely, these spots for deep thoughts are all over the house, like at the kitchen sink while I wash dishes, or around the bed as I change the sheets, or under the red bud tree outside as I pull seedlings. God wants to reveal God's great love for us everywhere.

It is *always* an acceptable time to wonder on God's great love for us. It is always a liminal time. Rev. Cindy Breed has this phrase on the tag of her emails: "Wait in quiet, loving attentiveness and see what God does next." That phrase has helped me with patience in these past days as my post #5 chemo-recovery has puttered along.

These days I'm not doing anything too quickly, so perhaps that is the blessing for me this year....just to sit in these incredible Bible texts, soak my feet in them and "wait in quiet, loving attentiveness and see what God does next."

Given a great idea
Posted Apr 5, 2012 10:51 a.m.

April 5, 2012, Maundy Thursday: I have great ideas. Of course in the recliner, this morning, I'm not coming up with any of them such that I have some sort of "evidence" of the great-idea-factory that I am, probably as a result of medications taken about 30 minutes ago with cranberry juice and peanut-butter-on-toast.

If I were to have had a great idea in the last, 72 hours, it would have looked something like this: Mom and Dad would have said to me "Hey, how about after Easter as you are past the most yucky time from chemo, if you ride along with us to go to see Eric and his family in Mississippi for a few days. You can just rest. We'll do the driving. It will be like a spa. Then we will get you back in time for chemo."

My response to their great idea was "I'm pretty sure that yes, I would like to do this." (Meaning: YES! I want to, but right know I feel so very yucky that I am having a hard time remembering what it might feel like to feel good again. And, two rounds ago I had nine days of feeling good, but the last time I only had five days of feeling good out of the twenty-one days in the round. So, yep, I'm a bit nervous.)

[Here is where the great idea factory, which is me, kicks in.] I remember very early on in our relationship with Dr. Mo that he said stuff like "Make your bucket list. Travel. Do the things that are important to you. We can work chemo and stuff around what ever is important to you." I appreciated this (early on) but clearly see that my bucket list has a whole layer over the top of it that looks like #1- get the cancer out of my body. #2 - repeat #1 if needed.
So, I think, "Hey. How about if just on this round, I wait four weeks instead of three weeks for chemo. After all, it would give me time to really rest up. I would sure feel a whole lot better going into chemo #6 if there was another week there between the trip to Mississippi and bellying up to the Chemo Bar." This is a great idea. Wow, do I have great ideas.

So, I will email Dr. Mo (copying the question to his nurses too) and ask him the question, relay all my rationale, and thank him for his good care of me and my family. That is what I did yesterday.

Late yesterday afternoon, Dr. Mo replied. "No, we cannot violate the study. Your lab results on before chemo determine whether or not you get treated that day. So, I'm afraid you will have to come as planned."
I cried. My bucket list still has #1 - get the cancer out of my body, but I'll tell you, there is a price to pay every time.

So, here it is, Maundy Thursday, one of my favorite days of the year. The Last Supper with Jesus and his disciples. Jesus washes his disciples' feet (John 13:1-20) and doing so, shows and tells them about love.

Today, I realize that I am still at that table. Judas is on one side of me, having just had a conversation about those odd deep dissolving stitches in my hip that looked like they were practically coming out through the top layers of skin but now seem to be staying there in place...unwanted...kind of like sin. Then I realize that Peter is on the other side of me. He is next in line to have Jesus wash his feet. Now, if I am a great idea factory, Peter is the mother-ship that delivers the factories to earth. He wants nothing to do with Jesus "serving him".....Peter knows that he is supposed to serve Jesus. That is just the way it is, and that is Peter's great idea.
Jesus says no, that isn't how it works. "You don't get to make that rule."
I completely identify with Peter. We absolutely love Jesus and think that our good ideas are great. Just listen to us tell about them!
But, Peter gets it. If he wants to be "a part" of whatever Jesus has going on, it has to be Jesus' way.
I get it. If I want to be "a part" of that clinical trial study for whatever length of time, it has to be the study founder and Dr. Mo's way. Oh, how we wish it were another.
The thing is, Dr. Mo has dedicated his life and work to healing people. The thing is, Jesus has already given his life and done the work. The wholeness Jesus offers comes through splashing in those baptismal waters and feasting on bread and wine and hearing the Word.

116

If I decide, or Dr. Mo decides, someday, that this study isn't the best thing for me, so be it. But for now, this odd-grace-great-idea-of-a-chemo-schedule is something that I might just wrestle with for a while longer.

Given a good washing...
Posted Apr 6, 2012 11:49 a.m.

April 6, 2012 Good Friday
Hiding what hurts.
Last evening I went to Maundy Thursday worship with a girl friend. After meditating on those scriptures for days, it wasn't surprising to me that about half way through worship I was searching my purse for a tissue. Of course the only one I could find was one covered with frogs wearing Santa hats. Through the whole worship I looked at that table set...bread and wine. I remembered my table mates, Judas and Peter, who shared my tendency to sin and to come up with great ideas beyond their calling.
(I've made my peace with my stitches which now I can see but not remove on my thigh. I've made my peace with my desire to have more of a break before the next chemo, and have decided that I will go to Mississippi with my folks, and just pray for safe travels and healthy fellow travelers and family members and know that my spirit will be renewed even if my body is tired as chemo round #6 starts. I will do this knowing that if my labs say I'm ready I will have chemo and if not, I won't. This time with my brother's family is every bit as healing for me as the chemo and dozens of medications I take over the course of three weeks.)
But you know who I met at worship? Jesus. Of course. Why should I be so surprised? After the graciously preached Word, there was an invitation to come forward to have one's feet washed. For the last eight years, I had been the one washing. This year I knew it was important to honor the gift that someone would give me, as they washed my feet.
When the pastor announced the "stations" for washing, I knew just where I wanted to go....to the spot where a mother (who is also a pastor) was washing and her little boy was drying. (I am going to guess his age as four years old.) I sat on the pew in front of where they knelt. My green sandals slipped off. First foot gently washed. First foot gently dried. I gave a

117

thumbs up to the drier as he looked up briefly for affirmation. The second foot -- the one with the bandaids on the big toe -- came along next to the drier. He got one look at those bandaids and shot me a look like "ohhhh....I respect your bandaids...." Then he extra-gently dried the top and bottom of that foot. No words were spoken. He just knew I needed the extra care.

Now, there is no place on me that really hollers out "cancer." Yet, in the drying of my feet, this caring young boy reminded me of Jesus, who, before going to the cross, took the time to know each of us -- feet and all -- and still said, "Yes. I will do this for you, just as you are."

That is the only reason this Friday is called Good.

Given a Saturday...
Posted Apr 7, 2012 12:13 p.m.

April 7, 2012 Holy Saturday: Why even have Holy Saturday? That is the question that woke me up this morning. As anyone who has ever hosted Easter breakfast/brunch/dinner -- you would know that you need time to go the the grocery store a few times, cook, clean, and make it all look effortless. That is a good 24 hours right there. Time to hunt for eggs is a more recent pastime.

The ancient church fathers (the church mothers were busy cooking and neglected to write down their equally great ideas) spent time thinking about this and had a few good reasons:

1) There just had to be some time in there to make sure Jesus was "really dead," otherwise the resurrection would look more like a magic trick or a lovely long healing nap.

2) Others said "read your First Peter, people, and remember that Jesus descended to the dead and spent the time overturning hell and preaching to the lost there, thus setting them free.

3) Still others said this was the perfect Sabbath for the Son of Man....resting from life, in death.

4) One of my favorite reasons comes in the Holy Saturday Gospel (Matthew 27:57-66) where the religious leaders (afraid that the whole raise-in-3-day thing would happen) suggested to Pilate that the tomb be sealed and guarded to prevent "tampering with the evidence." This

118

actually cracks me up. For the longest time I thought this "sealing" was sort of like creating a burping-Tupperware-like seal on the tomb to keep Jesus as fresh as possible until the ladies could come by with those spices after the Sabbath ended. Actually, the seal had more the effect of sealing wax on the back of an envelope; (1) making it impossible to get in/out without leaving evidence of tampering AND (2) making it in effect ILLEGAL to raise from the dead. No one was to break that seal...from the outside or the inside. (I have not listed the reason that pastors, the altar guild, and church musicians need a bit of a REST....hence the Saturday....that just goes without saying.)

I have another reason to add to this for "why Holy Saturday." Have you ever had someone very close to you die? Have you been a part of the early response to the death, and then had to not only call lists of people, but also visit the funeral home and make one zillion decisions, and then the church/pastor and make another zillion decisions, and then the florist and on and on. (Of course, I know people like myself who care very deeply about helping people through this time, but it remains some of the most difficult days in our lives).

There sometimes exists a time, maybe even a day, between the death and planning, and the visitation and funeral -- this is a type of "Holy Saturday"....time to wait, breathe, pray, wail, remember, hurt, laugh, cry. It is a crucial time to grieve. It is true that we await the resurrection, but right now (whenever that "now" is) we sit in the dust, tearing our sackcloth, refusing to eat.

I put into my "sack of collected Holy Saturday experiences," my pain. I had carefully planned a trip to Kohl's yesterday. This strategy included such things as waiting for certain medications to work through me so that I could drive, but not hurt so much that I couldn't walk; eat food (fish only on Good Friday for me) and have ample water available on the way to and from the shopping; have 20% off coupon for the appropriate day of sales; list the pants which no longer fit me (see weight gain noted on previous day); park strategically for minimal "out of store" walking; use time in store efficiently for maximum scanning and minimal searching for other sizes/colors.

This is what I did not plan: that I would be in so much physical pain (bones, muscles, head) from 4 to 10 p.m. that evening that I would do nothing much else beyond eat and sit in the recliner. This is quite frustrating. There is some bit of grief that this is so hard to do.

In my Holy Saturday "sack" I have put that grief, my sins, my overzealous planning/hoping, losses, having cancer, missing people in my congregation such that when I see them out and about it is very hard for me not to weep in their presence.

That "stuff" sits there today. The reality of the yuckiness of it is just there, not swept away by the all overriding glory, hope, grace and gift of the resurrection. For truly, the stuff in the sack has no power in the face of the resurrection. However, to not acknowledge it denies our shared humanity, and denies our need for the One who is spending today shaking up hell, and tomorrow will break Pilate's freshness seal on that tomb. The One who knows my feet, also knows what I've put in my Holy Saturday sack, and offers to carry it.

Given new life...
Posted Apr 8, 2012 8:22 a.m.

Alleluia! Christ is risen!

Hoping...
Posted Apr 11, 2012 12:19 a.m.

In my dining room, as well as in a few other places in my house, I have the word "HOPE" right out there where I can see it. Here at mom and dad's house, they have the Christmas card I sent them out on the kitchen counter....it spells "HOPE" as well.

Today, a dear seminary classmate, Pastor Julia Larsen Rademacher, posted something on facebook...and on the Liddy Shriver Sarcoma Initiative web site that says something about hope as well.

A while ago, Julia talked to me about the passion that she has developed for running. She's been preparing for a Half Marathon in Fargo, North Dakota, back in her home neck-of-the-woods. She asked if she could run a race and raise some funds for me. I told her that dear friends had already coordinated and held a huge fundraiser for my medical expenses. However, I also told her that sarcoma cancers are so rare that there are not the funds set aside for research on such rare diseases. I told her that when I was diagnosed, every single person who directed me to support for sarcomas (and there are over 100 of them) sent me to the Liddy Shriver Sarcoma Initiative site where 98% of the money they raise goes out in grants to people who are doing research on sarcomas. I said, that is where the money could go. I've looked at the site and saw some of the research that has been funded. I've also read about Liddy, a young woman who lived only 21 months with her sarcoma, and tried to make a difference for so many people. I know that Liddy Shriver and her family have made a difference for me.

Walking on air...
Posted Apr 16, 2012 11:25 p.m.

Home at last. I may not feel great, but this being home sure feels good after a week away. The time with family was so great. The prayers of the folks all along the way -- so appreciated. And then this: I got a call from my neighbor on the way home from Mississippi. "I'm just letting you know that the large tree behind your back fence lost a major limb -- it fell into your back yard...the garage is ok, the fence is ok, the house is ok, and it looks like you still have power, but the lines are down. I've called Mid American Energy Company (MEC) for you."
Maybe the next two days of neighbor, friend, tree removers, and Mid American Energy support wasn't supposed to be a welcome home gift, but I'm thankful it was.
Tonight we had Chinese food for supper. My fortune cookie read as follows: "Appreciate the caring people who surround you."
That I do.

Dear Lord, let this please be "over the hump" day

Posted Apr 21, 2012 11:16 a.m.

1 John 3:1-3 *See what love the Father has given us, that we should be called children of God, and that is what we are.......children of God is what we are....what we will be has not been revealed.*

Yesterday was every bit of 50 or more "hump days" all rolled into one. I would know that, as I have more than 50 camels. I remember some time back Dr. Mo saying whatever "way chemo went" would be the "way it would go." Yesterday, it did. I work (with the help of family and friends and doctors and nurses) to have it be as "better" as it can be. I try to do that. However, it is also just what it is. And, for Tuesday through Wednesday chemo, the next most immediate Friday afternoon and evening is my "hump-day."

This time I added one liter of normal saline fluids to the mix, given through my port over two hours at the infusion center in Moline. Because this is such a difficult time to drink enough, I hoped that would help. I did learn this....that the people there are very kind, that my friends who took me and stayed with me are champion foot massagers and tear driers. I think I wept for the first hour I was there. It seems like coming and going from Iowa City is just "what I do" now. I don't have to think about a cancer diagnosis as it is already established. But going to someplace new, even though well cared for, brought it all up again. One might think that after six to seven months now that this would not be new. Sigh.

This morning I was posed a question in a private message. All in all, these are hard to reply to, as I rarely have folks' email addresses. However, I always pray for those who ask for prayers. However, this particular question I want to answer. Maybe it will help me help others who are caring for me too.

I think that the gist of her question is something like "My dearest friend is entering the last phase of her life. She is so important to so many people and she is a child of God. I don't know how to care for her now. Can you tell me how to help her?"

Back when I was pastoring full time, I would talk to people in this stage about doing five things.

Be ready to say...and to hear her say:

I love you.

I'm sorry.

I forgive you.

Thank you.

Good bye.

I would add to that, that we cannot read minds. Yesterday, for me, telling me they loved me looked like passing me tissues, and bringing me food after food after food, trying to find something that wouldn't make me sicker. Saying they loved me sounded like grace at meal time. It was like texting me and telling me about their day. It was praying for me even when I didn't ask for it. It was reminding me that this hurdle could be hurdled a bit at a time. It was hearing funny stories. It was "being here now." It was being treated as a child of God, someone for whom Christ lived, died and rose again. That is an honor beyond measure and it may look a little different every day. Just ask. Your "continuing to be present" helps her have the courage to continue to be present as well.

Whatever
Posted Apr 23, 2012 11:04 p.m.

A few years ago Erica made me a framed cross stitch artwork of the word "whatever." I know that it is meant to be a bit more "in your face" sort of a word. We use it sometimes as a bit of a joke with a head shake and the shape of the thumb and first finger of each hand joined together in a big W on our foreheads when we don't want to say the word. I've left that word where I can see it.

I'm just about to enter week #2 of the three weeks of chemo. I'm beginning to feel like I have my "whatever" back. Meaning, my strength, my hope, my curiosity, my movement, my aches, my sense of humor, my "I can do this-- whatever this is." I don't have that so much that first week. The first week, I survive. At least I have so far.

I've had four or five different ideas of what to write about today. However, I'm so full of so many medications that I can't string together what those things might have been. Whatever! Yep. That works.

123

One thing I do remember, though, is this coming Sunday, "the Fourth Sunday of the Easter season," is thought of as Good Shepherd Sunday (John 10)....the one where Jesus speaks of doing whatever it takes -- laying down his life for his sheep. I am so incredibly thankful for that whatever. That's the one that counts. The rest are just "whatever."

Making a difference
Posted Apr 25, 2012 5:28 p.m.

Today is Blood Mobile Day in Pontiac, Illinois. My mom has been a coordinator of blood mobiles in my home town since the 1970s. On this day, a church that was signed up to sponsor the drive could not fulfill that commitment. Many circumstances came to bear and they just couldn't. Mom and Dad (her sidekick) and many of their friends who say "yes" when asked, made it happen on schedule. They know just when to move heaven and earth to get stuff done. For the dozens of people who will receive those blood products, it is the gift of life. I can't donate anymore, but I can be thankful for my folks and others who give that amazing gift.

I'm having a day where I'm wishing I could make my healing as simple as just "moving heaven and earth." That would be a direction, right? I know I'd have people who would help. Earlier today I took a call from a group of folks who are coordinating our lawn care. When I got off the phone I looked around for angels. I see them.

Today I decided that I could sit in the recliner no longer. I made cookies. To my credit, they are supposed to be "good for me." In the process I pushed myself to unload the dishwasher and wash the dishes from the cookie making. I wanted that to be just the thing that could lift my spirit. The cookies are good, but now I have spent two hours in the recliner "recovering" and I'm not sure it is going to work. So, maybe cookie baking isn't the cure-all that I hoped it would be.
Perhaps this is just a thinly veiled recruitment tool for the Red Cross or Mississippi Valley Regional Blood Bank. Maybe it is just a way to say, "Mom and Dad, you are doing a great job. Keep it up. I'm going to be just fine."

A letter...

Posted Apr 26, 2012 11:10 a.m.

I am grieving. Certainly we all have our griefs to bear. What I have been grieving this past month though, relates to the knowledge that I am not going to be able to return to ministry at Trinity Lutheran Church. I miss them and the ministry we share. This week I met with Bishop Gary Wollersheim (from the Northern Illinois Synod) and with Pastor Larry Conway (from Trinity). Both supported me with their presence, and with prayer, and in understanding of the direction I have chosen. I gave Pastor Larry a letter to be sent to the congregation. We decided on May 6 as the Sunday I would come to worship -- and to give and receive thanks in that setting.

This last month has been very difficult as I've prayed and prayed through this -- it is not good to grieve alone. And, as my pastor friends know, a first-call congregation holds a special place in the heart of pastors. Trinity is my first call.

Before you read the letter -- read this -- I have NO new news from my oncologist. I am staying the course. I have what Dr. Mo calls "stable disease" and am enrolled in a clinical chemotherapy trial that has no end date. If I were actively dying, I'm sure there would be a lot more people at my house and I would be coughing or hollering out for more pain meds or something. (My chemotherapy may kick the "get up and go" out of me for two-plus weeks, but it will not rob me of my sense of humor.)

April 25, 2012

Dear Brothers and Sisters in Christ of Trinity Lutheran Church,

Christ's mercy, grace and peace be yours, this day and every day.

*   In August of 2003, I gave God thanks for the precious call to serve in Christ's name as your associate pastor. It has been my honor to serve with you, with wonderful staff and with faithful leaders for over eight*

125

years. As a community of believers we have grown and served in significant ways. Being a part of your beginnings and endings, joys and sorrows, and resurrection hope has further shaped my faith and trust in God.

As you are aware, in September of 2011, I was diagnosed with sclerosing epitheloid fibrosarcoma. Since that time I have had two surgeries and undergone the first six of many rounds of chemotherapy in a clinical trial at the University of Iowa Hospital and Clinics. Your support, including prayers, help with the FUNdraiser, comments on my CarePages, countless cards and letters and more, have been significant in my wellness and signs of God's love to me and my family.

As you are also aware, I have been on disability during my illness. It had been my hope to receive treatment, get well, and return to ministry at Trinity. While my treatment and my hopes for cure continue, I am unable to work in my call as full-time pastor in a congregational setting.

With respect for the ongoing mission of Christ, I am removing my name from return to call at Trinity Lutheran.

Many years ago, my childhood Lutheran pastor gave me a "memory verse" which continues to give me strength -- Joshua 1:9 Be strong and courageous, neither afraid or dismayed, for the Lord your God is with you whereever you go.

At this point, I'm not "going" far. I will continue to live in the community. I will continue to have access to national-level sarcoma care in Iowa City. However, out of respect for future pastors and rostered leaders at Trinity, I will not return to perform pastoral acts such as baptisms, weddings, and funerals, nor will I perform formal acts of pastoral care. Do know, however, that I will continue to hold you in prayer and receive your prayers with thanksgiving as well. It is my hope that I will be able to serve in some ministry role in the future and will seek guidance from the synod should my physical condition allow this.

In this year of centennial celebration and thanksgiving, and always, "May the Lord bless you and keep you, May the Lord's face smile upon you and be gracious to you, May the Lord look upon you with favor and give you peace."

Your sister in Christ,

The Reverend Laura A. Koppenhoefer

126

...we have to go through it....
Posted Apr 27, 2012 7:39 p.m.

Although I am grieving as I figure out my call to ministry and cancer, I know we have been through tougher stuff. Likely most of you have as well. Likely you find that true from one grief to the next. Fortunately, it is not a contest!

So, here is my challenge -- I really like saying "Thank you" and "You're welcome" a whole lot better than I like saying "Goodbye." Maybe I am resisting on "Good-bye" because a little part of me feels like that is saying some sort of ultimate good-bye, and I am not ready for that. Right now, I would rather say "I'll see you at Target, or at HyVee, or at the movies."

However, I also know something about being ready to say "Hello" to somebody new in ministry. It is a whole lot better if first one has said "Goodbye" to the person who was there before. A good "Hello" is preceded by a good "Good-bye."

So, this is what I am going to work on: saying "Thank you" and "Good-bye" to Trinity as their associate pastor. Someone new will becoming who will need their "Hello."

Can this whole grief rigamaroll be avoided? You bet. People avoid staring straight at their griefs all the time. However, that isn't what we are called to be as individuals or in community. What will that sound like on May 6? -- I sort of imagine laughter and tears, singing and praying, telling stories and hearing God's story. And hugs (except if you have a cold/flu/fever as those hugs will have to wait for another day).

I could just spit.
Posted Apr 30, 2012 5:46 p.m.

So I did. I spit in the test tube.

I spit for a cause: the cause being researchers who want to learn more about the genetics of sarcoma.

But first....I registered on the www.23andme.com web site. I received the DNA testing kit in the mail. I registered my kit on line. I read the directions. (usually a good idea). I completed 30 minutes of health surveys on line while at the same time not eating or drinking for 30 minutes Then.....finally.....I spit into the test tube to fill up to the line (not counting the bubbles).I got it out to the mailbox only to find that the mail had already gone out for the day. -- Argh!

Well, tomorrow, this test will go in the mail. In four weeks or so, they will have some preliminary results. They will know things about me that I don't even know. Maybe, someday, something that they know about me and about thousands of other people with sarcoma, will help sarcoma (and other diseases) just go away.

What have I learned so far? The chemotherapy that I am taking wasn't even listed in the 25 possible chemotherapies for sarcoma. (It is too new.) The sarcoma that I have wasn't even listed in the 30 or so sarcomas listed. (There are over 100.) I am thankful that I do not have to depend on my disease for a sense of community...there aren't enough of us.

All the muscles....
Posted May 1, 2012 7:58 p.m.

Today is now night. I packed in my study at church with five helpers. Now I have 40% of my library packed and ready for seminarians and about 30% of the remaining books to pack.

Let's see, what else do I have? Aches. I didn't even lift a box, but just taking down book by book seems to have worked muscles in my chest that I have left rarely disturbed after I had my port inserted.

What else do I have? I have peace about a decision that I made this afternoon. Pastor Larry had graciously invited me to preach this Sunday. I had said that after my discussion with the Bishop, I thought that doing the Child's Word, presiding at Holy Communion, and offering the blessing would be just about right. Graciously, Pastor Larry offered it one more time, just in case I had changed my mind. As preacher, it is hard to say no to preaching. For 24 hours or so, I was thinking I might do it. Yet there is so much more to preaching than those minutes on Sunday. Just the 75 minute physical challenge of today was enough to remind me of my physical limitations. Sunday, even being in worship, let alone leading parts of it, will be a challenge. I don't want me "looking like I'm about to fall asleep or about to keel over" to be a distraction from the joy of our shared worship. I've got peace about this, and that feels better than any other place on me.

Thankful...
Posted May 5, 2012 12:00 a.m.

This noon hour I went back to church. I've been there over the noon hours for the last three days with four or five friends each day. With their help, all of my books are packed, and the desk and the filing cabinets are emptied. I did a lot of sorting. A lot of sorting. The trip down ministry-memory-lane revealed that ministry has continued to evolve to meet the needs of the gathered community and to develop and reflect the ministry gifts of the community as well. While I'm not thankful for the reason I am emptying my office, I'm thankful for the reminder that good things have happened in these years, and I'm confident that the Spirit continues to breathe through the church when it gathers and when it is sent to serve.

This evening, I cleaned out the refrigerator. That task has been my mom's for many months. She really does have some great refrigerator cleaning skills. Tonight, however, I sorted through that fridge like a woman on a mission. I don't think there is any deep similarity between old groceries and old files. However, the deep feeling of thankfulness that came over me as I cleaned it out was similar. I was thankful doing a simple household task -- and to feel pretty good while doing it.

Endings....middles.....beginnings
Posted May 7, 2012 12:06 p.m.

I am still overwhelmed by the love, prayers, and care of the community of Trinity Lutheran. I also don't know if I have ever hugged that many people in one day before! Seeing those wonderful faces brought memories of baptisms and weddings, funerals and crisis, meals and projects and more.

After the first 15 minutes or so of embraces after each worship I was crying enough that we could have collected the water for a baptism! Oh my. I can't say that I enjoyed the eight hours of aching that happened later in the day, but for the opportunity to experience the love and care of that community, and to be able to say "Thank you" and "Good-bye" to my former call, I am truly grateful.

The experience has me wondering about beginnings and endings and middles. While yesterday was an ending, I found that so much of my sorrow was because we were very certainly in the middle of so many things together. I am thankful that my not being there didn't mean the end of those things. My hope in the ministry has been that when people looked to me, that they would see me pointing to Jesus.

Today begins my preparation for Chemo Round #7, yet I am in the middle of my healing. This is also national Nurses' Week, so I will thank my nurses for helping me through yet another middle.

Chemo #7, a quick update
Posted May 8, 2012 7:44 p.m.

The day started off right on schedule, however slowed down significantly as we got here to Iowa City. The great news is that my port worked *perfectly*!

Dr. Mo and Regina (the study nurse) are preparing me for three weeks from now when I will get my twelve week scans. He has said that he might stop my chemo if he sees stuff stable in my lungs and sees ongoing struggles with my liver. The liver toxicity might be reason enough to stop this chemo and take a rest. He did not say if he could start me back up if I took a break, so we have a lot to learn.

A new day...
Posted May 13, 2012 9:49 a.m.
It is Mother's Day...and I am:
1) thankful in both directions....for my mom, grandmothers and daughters
2) beginning to feel better
All this is worth celebrating...

Disruption
Posted May 15, 2012 9:20 a.m.

Last fall I started a small collection of books. Each one had something to do with cancer and people who had lived through the "experience." Without exception, I started reading each one of them and stopped before I was 60% of the way through. I'm not sure why I did. Maybe I realized that I wanted company on the journey, but didn't feel compelled to "do the journey" the same way that others had. Or, perhaps I was worried that they had won, and I wouldn't.

In the many months since I've read lots of books -- sometimes ones suggested by Erica. She loves good books and has a keen eye for plot and such. Then this weekend I got ahead of her listed suggestions and went back to a book that I had started in October -- *Disrupted: On Fighting Death and Keeping Faith*, by Julie Anderson Love, a former Presbyterian pastor who survived an extremely malignant brain tumor. Her aggressive treatments were called "disruption." She lives on the west coast and got her treatments at Oregon Health Sciences University Hospital, where I got my master's in nursing. She survives, yet as I learned last night, lost about 90% of her hearing in the treatment. I would rather lose my hair.

As I read now, she is relating her experiences to Job's life, as in Job in the Bible (in the chapter titled "No," pages 95 -107).
As I continued, she related her decisions about treatment, and the wrestling there-of, to God/the Angel's wrestling with Jacob (in the chapter titled "Limping," pages 133-145).
Then late last night she shared how alone she felt in her decisions (even with loving people around her and great doctors), wondering with the Psalmist, and Jesus... "My God, my God, why have you forsaken me?" (returning to the chapter "No" and a reflection on Psalm 22).
I have wondered the same.

This morning, in the quiet of the house, I wonder how I write these days. In the same 24 hours that find me wresting along familiar paths with others who know Christ and who also know illness. I am fixin' to be

131

"disrupted." The chemo process-routine-argh-fest is going up for review in two weeks. I am fixin' to be re-scanned and my plan re-evaluated and what I know so far, re-directed. I am spending a lot of time on the wrestling mat right now. (That, or, my hip just hurts again because of an expected weather change, or, because it is still trying to spit out stitches.)

Last night, as I watched Dancing with the Stars, I tried a bit more of my "fancy washcloth knitting." It didn't go so well. I was having a hard time tracking rows. I re-counted. I had repeated a pattern that wasn't supposed to be repeated and I was lost. I stopped and re-started several times. Finally, I tore out three rows to get back to a place where I knew what I was doing. Then, I set it down. There will be times for the "tough knitting" when I am tracking more clearly.

Perhaps this week it is enough to focus on what is here right now. Right in front of me. "Be here now."

A new view
Posted May 16, 2012 10:58 a.m.

Two years ago I removed the wall paper in my dining room and painted it a wonderful blue. It took me six months to put one thing on the wall. (By this, I mean have my dad hang something on the wall in a place of my choosing.) There are risks to putting nails in lath and plaster 80-year-old walls. My personal nightmare looks something like the nail going in and the surrounding 10-foot area crumbling to the floor in something like dust and tears. The first print that went up was a wonderful Amish woodcut of flowers in a basket. It had hung in my Grandma and Grandpa Harding's home for years.

Last fall, picture #2, a striking photo of a sunflower, photographed by my cousin Sheryl Svoboda, "made the wall." So far so good. Two major areas have remained unadorned. Waiting.

Then a few weeks ago, I boxed up my office at church, bringing home my wall art. Three things I especially missed seeing each day -- a large cross that my brother and Katherine gave me, some contemporary art with the reminder from scripture that we can do all things though Christ who strengthens us, and, the picture I had taken of Gamal, the camel, on his journey with all the other camels on an old storefront step in Jerusalem. With Dad's help, all three "made the walls" on Monday. With dad's help I'm reminded that there is beauty everywhere.

Things that help, Part 9
Posted May 17, 2012 11:05 a.m.

I am just past week one post chemo and find that the slope from Point A (feeling absolutely horrible) to Point B (feeling lousy with aching, headaches and fatigue) is a slippery one. I get a sort of indignant voice in me that speaks out something like "Point A is done and good riddance. You deserve a 'pass' on Point B -- so claim it! You go girl!" FYI-- this voice has no authority, and her enthusiastic technique does not work. In the absence of any help from this voice, my "whiny" voice shows up way too easily. This is not good. I may not remember everything from my childhood, but I do remember that my parents invested 15-20 years of their lives in me *not* being a whiner.

So, today (again) I will ignore the ineffective enthusiastic voice, and I will silence the whiner voice.

Today I choose to lift up the "things that help" right now, today, in thanksgiving to the One whose voice I strive to hear above all others.

1) *Kitchen Table Wisdom* by Rachel Naomi Remen, MD....which I was not ready to read when it arrived many weeks ago, but is truly a good companion now.

2) Foot massages

3) Peanut butter on toast

4) The swing on the back deck

5) The piano in my living room

6) My daughters who carried the book shelves to the living room as well

7) The people who planted seeds many many weeks ago and are tending those things at nurseries until I feel well enough to do the shopping I love to do

8) Both of my daughters having jobs

9) That I am enjoying writing.....even more than knitting, right now

10) That my mat carriers pray for me....and at my request will likely help me by praying for me to drink more water.... more water would help, I think

11) That I am not alone on the journey

Some action from the front row
Posted May 18, 2012 10:11 a.m.

In the summer of 1999, Rod and I sold our house on Jenny Lind Drive in Normal, Illinois, took our daughters to Disney World, temporarily moved in with Rod's mom for the summer, and I started Summer Greek at Wartburg Seminary in Dubuque. On the first day of Summer Greek, I sat down in the front row of desks with Beth, Jon, and Julia. My Greek translational skills are pretty rusty, but I still count the people from the front row as my friends. Tomorrow, Julia is running her first half-marathon in Fargo, North Dakota, in my honor, to raise money for sarcoma research funded by the Liddy Shriver Sarcoma Initiative.

I am in a very supportive Facebook group for people with sarcoma and their families. It is one of the groups that led me to the resources available from the Liddy Shriver Sarcoma Initiative. On the Facebook site, on any given day, people are expressing frustration over lost friends and lost limbs, rejoicing that treatment is working or grieving that there is no more treatment available. They speak the truth about the side effects of treatments and rattle off names of chemotherapies and surgeries that they or the people they love have endured for months, or years. It is the kind of community that we wish all communities were like, but we wish this community could just go away, because sarcoma cancer would be no more.

Calling all saints....

Posted May 21, 2012 11:37 a.m.

This morning, my scripture reading comes in preparation for next Sunday....Pentecost -- the "birthday" of the church. I started my reading with Acts 2:1-11. And, what did I find? The same sorts of problems that my family has in remembering "who was there."

I never thought much about that list of the nations represented in Jerusalem for the festival prior to seminary, except if I had been challenged to be a lector for the day. However, that old list has me wondering in a different way today. I've known for a dozen years or so that all of those nations listed there couldn't possibly have been in Jerusalem then. Two of them, the Medes and the Elamites were "extinct" and had been for 500-600 years. Now if I were prepping for preaching I would have lots of directions to go here. However, today I'm just trying to sort out family videos in chronological order and keep the clutter contained in my living room.

I will make these observations though: Vocally, right now, I sound just like my mom did at age 50. The knitting needles I'm using now are likely the same ones my Grandma Davis used to knit a ball that baby Erica played with in Beaverton, Oregon 23 years ago. That the Harding family gathered for Father's Day at the farm in 1994 was quite excited to know if my sister-in-law had gone into labor yet with their first son, that son who when smiling in a video at five months of age, smiled with the same smile he has now as he finishes his junior year in high school --- handsome and engaging. That Rod taught 2-year-old Sarah to raise both hands in the air above her head and shout "Touch down!" I'm pretty sure she still has that skill.

Truly, I think that all of us are all here all the time. It is no more surprising to say that the Medes and Elamites were there than it is to say that you can taste my Grandma Harding's baking in my cookies. We give some of our selves to all who follow us. We can't remember the years because it doesn't matter. The fact that we are here or were here, that is what matters. The fact that the same Spirit blows through us -- through the generations-- that matters. The fact that love remains, that matters.

The day of the great garden experiment
Posted May 23, 2012 11:49 a.m.

Bit by bit plants have been planted around the deck and yard. So far, most things have stayed planted. By "staying planted," I mean "have not been dug-up and used for rabbit/squirrel/chipmunk/snake/groundhog/bird lesson in 'how to really irritate Laura.' I have listed all the furry, winged, or reptilian creatures of the yard as possible culprits because I have not been witness to the "digging up." If I was a witness, surely I would have prevented it. I think we all know that the rabbit/squirrel/chipmunk set is most likely guilty.

That is the 2012 backdrop for this, the day of the great garden experiment. The rest of the information you need follows:

1) The Koppenhoefers, when living in Normal Illinois, were able to grow large sunflowers quite successfully. One year, our Christmas card was the four of us standing in the garden by our 13 1/2 foot bloomer.

2) That experience has left us with practically impossibly high standards for our own sunflower growing future success.

3) The previous two times I have tried to grow sunflowers in this Rock Island yard, they were beautifully planted in a row, parallel to two varieties of zinnias. All emerged from the ground. All got to the 4-leaf stage. All of the zinnias were left alone. All of the sunflowers were eaten to the ground. (See previous list for culprits.)

4) I have friends who have grown sunflowers locally.

5) These friends may or may not have the same culprits living in their yard.

6) Some of these friends are committed to helping me grow sunflowers. (None of my friends have been committed....I just want to be clear about that.)

7) Sunflowers are the flowers for sarcoma.

Today Stacie and Penny are coming to my house to create a "safe place" for sunflowers to grow in my yard -- an eight foot square protective "play pen" for sunflowers...and the 2012 sunflower saga begins.

Days by the numbers
Posted May 24, 2012 7:11 p.m.

As a math teacher's daughter, this seems as good a day as any to count my blessings:

1,325 - The number of dollars raised by Pastor Julia Rademacher for sarcoma research! Hurray!

101 - The approximate dollars raised per mile in the half marathon by Julia.

3 - The number of days it was before she says she was really sore.

3 - The number of rows of sunflowers planted in the newly constructed sunflower "playpen."

34 - The number of boxes of books and office stuff delivered today from Trinity.

9 - The number of boxes of books emptied so far.

2 - The number of carts of plants purchased by Penny and me at Wallace's Garden Center.

30 - The approximate number of yards that a Wallace cart, one third full of our plants, rolled downhill away from my vehicle in the parking lot.

2-fast - The approximate speed of a Wallace cart.

1 - The number of guys on motorcycles leaving the Wallace parking lot at the same speed as our cart.

1 -The number of guys who stopped their motorcycle and helped Penny scoop up the plants

ALL - The number of plants that survived the "spill"

Two updates
Posted May 25, 2012 3:00 p.m.

(1) The size of the fencing (meaning the hole size) equals the size of the chipmunks. It appears they like sunflower seeds. (2) My watering of the plants/seeds last evening, combined with making sure the rain gauge was empty, and the general cloudiness, did not in fact make it rain. I'll try harder next time.

The day before
Posted May 28, 2012 10:49 a.m.

"Why is there a frog on my tea box?" Really? My tea box is talking to me? I keep reading. Lipton tells me that my tea has been grown on a Rainforest Alliance Certified tea farm. That is what I read around the little frog that sits in the middle of a seal. Well, now I feel better about my tea, of course, but the question remained, "Why is there a frog on my tea box?"

I think this is a day, and tomorrow will be another day, when the best possible thing to do is to fully rely on God....Father, Son and Holy Spirit. That's all. (And drink water, of course.) Tomorrow will be a long day in Iowa City. I have my labs drawn in the morning. My CT scan and MRI follow in the afternoon. Then, I don't meet with Dr. Mo until 4:00 p.m., or later. That is when he will make a decision on my chemotherapy.

Given my tea box experience, I plan to look for and find God in unexpected places.

No more chemo for now
Posted May 29, 2012 10:22 p.m.

It is after 9 p.m. and we are finally home. As I suspected after chemo #7, Dr. Mo stopped the Trabectadin chemotherapy. I am thankful for the break, and ready to feel better for a while. We are all tired from the long day, but certainly I am feeling better than if I had started chemo at the end of it. So, this is what I know so far:

1) Complete scan results are not in yet but Dr. Mo did know a few things.
2) No new tumors in my lungs. This is great.
3) The tumors that are in my lungs are ever so slightly larger. Not as great, but the tumors are still pretty small.
4) There is no growth in the former tumor area in my hip.

138

5) The fibroids that had been in my uterus for years are smaller (He kind of said this as an aside after we had talked about everything else for about 45 minutes.)

6) He will have final results of my scans in 48 hours. I have to return next week for an EKG and a MUGA scan (nuclear medicine scan of my heart).

7) Dr. Mo suspects that six to seven rounds of this chemotherapy is just as effective as many more rounds, although the research does not say that definitively.

8) My liver values have been steadily increasing with each round of chemotherapy, and the amount of medicine that I need to keep my GI system in check, plus all the pain, means that it is time to give my body a rest.

9) I will have scans in six to eight weeks. Dr. Mo thinks that my tumors are very slow growers and at this point I think he is unlikely to restart chemo until the tumors do something like double in size. Whether that happens in six months or a year or more, he wants my body to heal well so that my body will tolerate whatever chemo he thinks is best.

10) Dr. Mo is very hopeful that my hip will heal better now. He said that six months would not be an abnormal healing time for that surgery and I only had eight weeks before I started chemo. Nothing really heals while on chemo.

There may be more than ten details, but that is what I can remember for now. Let's get healing.

A nature walk with the Trinity
Posted Jun 1, 2012 9:47 a.m.

Yesterday I spent a lot of time checking my email to see if Dr. Mo had sent me anything yet. At about supper time he sent me the radiologist's reports of my MRI and CT scans, which repeated what he had said on Tuesday....a little growth in the lungs. I seem to notice that when I have days like that -- where my focus is a "worried focus" -- God offers something big, something I can't miss. Yesterday it was the rain. We really needed the rain here and it came slowly and steadily. By the time it quit in the late afternoon we had an inch. As I hoped, the new plantings are well watered....and so am I. Water is such a baptismal remembrance for me that when I think of looking back outside over the yard, I hear the phrase "Child of God" again and again.

That helps me. For when it seems that everything might change, God says one thing never changes. I love you.

So when the rain was almost stopped, I checked the rain gauge. I had to be ready with the rainfall amount -- in case someone called and wanted to know! Then, when the rain was over, I did a crop inspection....or rather God and I did a crop inspection....The Creator was just beaming....things in bloom and green. The Son walked along side me for company. And the Spirit came with to give me peace, as I learned that the chipmunk had made it into the play pen and knocked over one of the sunflower seedlings; "someone" had dug up an impatiens; "someone else" had chopped off two-thirds of the coral bells bloom stems, and the robins had started another nest in the wreath by the front door. The playpen of sunflowers was left as is; the impatiens re-planted; the coral bells brought in to a pretty vase, and, the wreath relocated to inside the garage. When I removed the last two nests from the wreath in the early spring, I thought that the birds understood I was uncomfortable having a nest twelve inches from my head as I came out the front door. (Note: I am bird-phobic.) However, when their newest nests got wet in the gutters in the rain, I think they decided to see if I was more tender-hearted. Me, not so much tender hearted related to front-porch-nesters.

I am so thankful that it is spring/summer. I can be outside and putter around in the garden with God. I am reminded that the world is so much bigger than my momentary troubles and issues, and that God's creativity and love are boundless.

What could get better?

Posted Jun 2, 2012 11:07 a.m.

This morning I read my friend, Rev. Janet Hunt's blog (Dancing with the Word) for my devotion. She does some wondering about Nicodemus (John 3), and I have too.

Last evening a seminary friend and his wonderful wife visited. He was reminiscing about the days when he drove his kids and ours in the car pool to elementary school in Dubuque. One of the "features" of his car was his singing crazy songs. One of those was an absolutely ridiculous song that he made up. He asked if the girls or I remembered any of the songs and I promptly sang every word of that ridiculous song. Even he remarked on my accuracy. However, in our conversations over glasses of water in the living room, I could lose my place in conversation or forget something that I know I knew earlier in the day. I have come to call the phenomena "chemo brain" as do some others with similar experiences. I miss my pre-chemo "youth."

In her blog, Janet wonders about Nicodemus, who has grown old, and who wonders how one can be born again, or born from above as Jesus says. I can almost feel Nicodemus' mind wander quickly to "what hurts" or "what doesn't work the way it used to" or simply "what if I could start over?" Is it that kind of born again?

These days I wonder what will feel better. I don't have nausea. That is so good to be free of. When will the other pains and shortness of breath be relieved? Will the chemo brain go away? Dr. Mo says I will begin to feel better. He emailed me yesterday to tell me that I am "off of the study" because my tumors grew greater that 20%. As he said, because the tumors are so small (about 1 cm each), it is not hard to have greater than a 20% growth. That would only be two millimeters growth each, after all. Oh, to be born again....

But Jesus says that the birth he is talking about isn't birth from back in the womb, it is from above, it is from the Spirit. It is a birth that is a new gift every day. Even in the midst of longing for memory and breath and some physical things to improve, I have received countless gifts of renewal for my spirit....visits from local friends, time with my daughters, beautiful plants growing in my yard, the gift of rain, cooler days, uplifting and challenging blogs from a friend, visits from pastor friends who are passing through, even an upcoming visit from one of my sisters-in-law. Yes, every single day there have been gifts of renewal for my spirit from the Spirit. I don't have to wait for it to get better, it is made better before my asking. This kind of birth reminds me that we have already entered kingdom of God. I can see it all around me already.

Fixin' to get ready...
Posted Jun 4, 2012 11:38 p.m.

Tomorrow morning (Tuesday) is an early one as Dee (Rod's sister) and I head to Iowa City for some follow-up heart tests (a "MUGA"---a radiologic test similar to an echocardiogram, and an ECG). These are routine, and called for because I am leaving the study. Later in the day I will be headed to Pontiac to stay with my folks. On Friday I will head with them to Mississippi. I think a little time on the lake with family will be a great place to heal.

Remembering why to memorize
Posted Jun 6, 2012 12:52 p.m.

I'm at my folks' home in Pontiac. It's so beautiful here...a lovely home built in wooded land that had only ever been pasture. Wonderful neighbors in people, flora, and fauna (with the exception of the deer when they eat the hostas or the newly planted trees). It is a good place to rest up, heal up, eat good food, and get ready for that trip to Mississippi.

In the quiet house this morning, I found that the second lesson for this coming Sunday looked familiar, and it was; I memorized it years ago:

2 Corinthians 4:16-18...*16 So we do not lose heart. Even though our outer nature is wasting away, our inner nature is being renewed day by day. 17 For this slight momentary affliction is preparing us for an eternal weight of glory beyond all measure. 18 Because we look not at what can be seen but at what cannot be seen; for what can be seen is temporary, but what cannot be seen is eternal.*

I've shared that at the bedside of countless people, and in these past months, especially on days when I couldn't focus to read, or remember what I had just read, I said it again, for myself. The stuff that I "see" on me like scars, or even in me via scan results can be quite distracting. The gift of daily renewal (or even moment to moment renewal) and the promise of the eternal helps to recenter me. However, it is not just this scripture (or hymn/song, or creed, or whatever) that can be renewing. I am continually thankful for the gift of having memorized some of my favorite scripture. And, I will say that that is a gift that does not disappoint. Even if I try to get something memorized and it doesn't stick like I want it to, I still learn so much from the repetition.

One year in seminary we were required to memorize Luther's Small Catechism -- The Apostles' Creed, 10 Commandments, Lord's Prayer, the Sacraments, and Confession, with the meanings. In my case and many others it meant re-memorizing, because we had done so in junior high or earlier. However, English has been updated over the years and we had to learn the updated version. I did pretty well until the meaning of the last three petitions of the Lord's Prayer. It was as if my memory card was full. So, I picked a familiar hymn tunes and set the meanings to those tunes. Now, ten years later, the parts I remember the most are the ones I set to music.

I've found that in these last months there were times that the last thing I would be able to do would be to remember new things, even scripture. Pain or nausea or medications or "whatever" messed so many things up. However, what I had set to memory years ago was available to me immediately. I am thankful to have made that investment.

Something I miss...
Posted Jun 7, 2012 11:19 a.m.

I was reading a column by a pastor in Minnesota about presiding at weddings. She claims that pastors either love to do this, or they don't. Likely she is right. Personally, I love to do this. In years that I was especially busy with weddings, I did miss a significant amount of time with my family, but I still enjoyed the six or so hours spent premaritally with couples and the time of their rehearsal and wedding. As friends packed up my office with me, I was reminded that for a few years of pastoral transition at Trinity, I had as many as ten weddings a year for two or more years. Now it has been almost a year since my last wedding.

My daughters tease me because I watch reality TV. I do love the shows with dancing, singing, cooking, and bridal fashion. Actually, ministry provided plenty of reality, as has my own life.

I think the main reason I love working with premarital couples is for the opportunity to speak God's reality to them....especially to those who have not heard it lately, or ever. The church (broadly) and Christians (broadly) are often their own worst enemies; forgetting to preach/demonstrate the grace that they have been so freely given. Sitting across from someone in a premarital session who was bullied in some church somewhere, or whose honest questions were seen as lack of faith or hatred of the church; well, sitting across from those people would lead me to offer heartfelt apology for that church in that time, and a vision of God's great love that remained present and available right there, right then.

At every step of the "wedding" process, there was the opportunity to offer God's welcome to that couple and to those who they knew...or those who at least came by for a good party. For many folks, seeing a woman presider might have been a first-time experience. So, I hoped, out of curiosity at the very least, they might just listen and hear something about God's love or about hope or about new life or about healing in a new way. And, maybe then their "most recent" experience with a church might be a positive one. Maybe they might get a glimmer that there is so much more to marriage than that day, and the dress, and the aisle runner. Maybe they might get a glimmer of this God who truly is present in sickness and in health, in plenty and in want.

Life is reality where the Spirit still shows up every single day, right where we need her.

Joy is....

Posted Jun 10, 2012 8:07 p.m.

...good vacation food...countless rounds of Uno and Mexican Train Dominos...telling family stories...breakfast times that last 3 hours...good sleeping (with an occasional nap)...reading good books...watching my mom water ski...seeing the smooth lake water after an afternoon storm...being Aunt Laura

Trust and blossom
Posted Jun 12, 2012 1:03 a.m.

Today Mom, Dad, and I, along with my brother and sister-in-law and their two sons and two daughters left the lake house and returned to their home in New Albany, Mississippi. We got to watch my (high school-aged) nephews play basketball and it was well worth the trip to do so. The most amazing look and sound of the day came from my youngest niece at the basketball game. Full of joy and love and trust, she called to my brother, "Dad!" He hears that every day and loves it, I am confident. All of their children are loved. Their daughters are newer to our family. It has been three years since they arrived at their home to be fostered, and about a year and a bit since their adoption. (The girls are now five and seven.)

One of the images of baptism that I appreciate is one of adoption by God. All the baptized are Children of God....not nieces, or nephews, or second cousins once removed; children. The look of love and trust in my niece's face is one that models for me the look that I strive to have toward God. She is confident her Daddy and Mommy love her, and they do. In their parents' love, all four of them blossom.

Through this "many month" ordeal with cancer, I have had many grown up conversations with God. (It is a part of our relationship. God is honest with me and I am honest with God.) I bring up this grace-filled look on my niece's face, because I think it is a memory that can help me remember God's love of me and my family on those days when I over-focus on other things (like scans and pills, scars and pain) rather than on God's promises of love and trustworthiness, forgiveness and healing. I see the Spirit working through my niece, to help me understand God's love for me and all of us. I am quite confident that she loves her daddy, because he loved her first. So it is with God.

Feeling "in-between"
Posted Jun 16, 2012 4:02 p.m.

I can remember many times in my life when I have felt "in-between" people -- as a communicator, a negotiator or an advocate. For the last few days, I'm feeling "in-between" times. Times like between scans. Between feeling lousy and feeling better. Between the delivery of all of my office stuff to my house and having it all put away. Between birth and death.

After having months and months of focus on surgery or chemotherapy or scans or whatever, I'm left wondering what I do "in-between" times. At 50, I feel it is too early to only pay medical bills, knit or crochet, and watch the Hallmark Channel (although I am getting to be a bit of an expert on recent episodes of *The Waltons* and *Little House on the Prairie*).
So, I've decided to look for direction. This is what I did at other in-between times in my life, anyway. Today I visited with my spiritual director to get that process restarted. I also moved the Jesus doll from the sunroom to the living room. I figured that the cross pictures were great, but some times seeing Jesus reminds me to talk to him. Someone dear gave me a picture of Jesus that I use for that purpose in my bedroom.
I guess that all of life is "in-between" time, and it's not like I haven't done some sort of spiritual wandering and wondering before. All of it is worth praying about....God would like that conversation as much as I would.

Wandering, fear and faith
Posted Jun 20, 2012 10:53 a.m.

For the last two days I have been wandering around -- mainly around the house and the yard. I do a bit on projects here there. The kitchen and living room are clean and free of boxes, but the rest of the place has been up for grabs. Outside, some of the landscaping has had a few weeds pulled, but if the weeds aren't taller than the featured plants, they will likely get to stay for a while.

146

I promise myself that I will clear the sunroom of boxes today. Making that promise means that I have to make some sort of decision about what to keep in a box, what to keep out. What to offer to another good home, and what to recycle or throw away. I've gone through the books and done this already, but now it is time to go through my frog collection.

I can't go through this stuff without becoming aware of the fear I have during this three-month-time-in-between-scans. How do I put things away? With confidence that they will be needed again for ministry in a church? With the thought that if they are away that I don't have to address my fears? With a fear that I will never open this box again? After all, the fears have nothing to do with my stuff, it is about my life.

As I un-pack and re-pack, moving slowly around, I wonder why I fear at this time, of all times. I have already survived two surgeries, a port insertion, seven 24-hour chemos and one additional hospital stay. Wouldn't that have been the time to fear? Those were certainly the times most like the Gospel for this week from Mark (4:35-41) where Jesus, tired from a day of preaching, asks to be taken across the Sea of Galilee. While on the ride, Jesus falls asleep. A storm comes up and the seas threaten to overtake the boat. The disciples are afraid and wake Jesus up. "Hey, Jesus! What is this with being 'asleep at the wheel'? It's like you don't even care about yourself or us! What's up with that?" (....paraphrased by me) Then Jesus rebukes the wind and speaks to the seas. Done. A dead calm.
In the last many months (since September 2011), Jesus and I have had several "Are You Asleep At the Wheel?" conversations.

It was easy for me to imagine Jesus and his best buddies in that boat with the wind and the seas soaking them all. I felt like I was in the boat with them on many occasions. Now, though, it seems that I can come up with questions for "Napping Jesus" when stuff is too calm. What is going on in my lungs while I can't see? Is the nerve damage in my hip going to reverse or at least feel better? Will I go back to parish ministry? Will I see my own grandchildren?

Yep, these are exactly the times that I figured would come again. This is why I put the Jesus doll in the living room, just to my right as I sit in the recliner. I see him each time I reach for my glass of water. Water that is not stormy. Water that heals. Water that, with the Word, makes me a Child of God. Water that grows God's creation in ways beyond my imagining. Water that connects me to the greater community. And, then I am reminded that "it's not all about me." It is not surprising that I have fears. Who wouldn't? Who doesn't? However, the boat I'm in is the same one Jesus is in. He was in it when the seas were stormy. He's in it still while they are calm. This is faith. This is trust. I may still fear what lies ahead, but I have trust in the One who walks with us all.

Oh give thanks to the Lord...
Posted Jun 21, 2012 9:40 a.m.

Psalm 107 begins this way ...
O give thanks to the LORD,
for he is good;
for his steadfast love endures forever.
Let the redeemed of the LORD say so, those he redeemed from trouble,
And gathered in from the lands,
from the east and from the west,
from the north and from the south (or, sea).
Yesterday as I wrote, I was preparing to "take on" my sunroom and the boxes that had collected there, out of the way of most traffic, but clearly in sight of everyone. In that great pile, were over 110 frogs, most of them given to me over the years. As I began my work for the day, I saw them as a burden, "taking up room." They were most definitely a tool for ministry, and, that particular ministry was concluded. What should I do with them now? Then I started sorting them; all of the Little frogs -- from lights to keychains, soap to snacks, rings to wind-up toys -- all were assembled on the dining room table. Then the stuffed frogs took their place on the sofa. After an hour or so of sorting and photographing, I realized I was playing.
I began to realize that I liked my collection just as it is and that I wanted to keep it. Yes, it still reminds me to Fully Rely on God (FROG). The little frogs then went into two pretty boxes (to be retrieved easily for whatever

148

purpose) and many of the stuffed ones the same. After I had finished photographing the frogs on the table and those on the sofa, I began to realize how many more I had around my house: planters, pillowcases, mugs, a motion detector, salt and pepper shakers, great t-shirts, pads of paper, and countless stickers.

They serve as a joyful reminder that I have ministry to perform every day. We all do for one another. I guess I had better hop to it.

A video reminder
Posted Jun 22, 2012 10:11 a.m.

After posing the frogs for their photos the other day, I began to realize how many "frog things" I had not gotten in the picture. So, for the next day or so, I went around taking pictures of the frog stuff "in their natural environment": the frog on the stick in the flowers in the garden, the frog blankets on the recliner, frog planters with plants in them, frog wind chimes hanging outside, frog salt and pepper shakers in the kitchen, and frog "motion detector" -- where ever I want it!

As I looked through my collection, I remembered that several of the frogs are "international" -- the frog instrument from Thailand, the green porcelain one from South America, a little green one from Germany (I purchased), and one from Austria and one from Ghana from the youth at church who remembered me on their travels. These frogs remind me of the broad embrace of God....all around the world.

Then, last night when I went to bed, I looked at my pillow cases -- yep, frog ones, made for me as my chemo journey began, by my sister-in-law, Dee. I've been sleeping on them for months, and I didn't think of them when I took all those pictures. That's just the way it is some times, there are people and things around me all the time to support and encourage me, yet I don't always remember they are there. Rev. Randy Willers, my "ordination brother" (ordained in the same worship service at synod assembly in 2003) mentioned a book that could be helpful to me, even offering to bring me one now, called *Jesus, Remember Me: Words of Assurance From Martin Luther*. I know it is a good book, as he gave me a copy after Rod died and I have shared other copies with people over the past several years. However, I had forgotten it was on the shelf until he mentioned it again.

I picture the people who gave me frogs. I smile in gratitude. Their thoughts and prayers are signs of God's graciousness and constant presence, as well.

An early morning report
Posted Jun 26, 2012 10:27 a.m.

Rock Island - An early morning survey of crops in a local yard reveals that some bandit - known locally as the "Furry Avenger" - has continued his/her mission of destruction. A perilous climb to the heights of the deck table came with the reward of a tasty treat -- one half of one pink-flowering begonia plant. This comes after the previous day's loss of one of three Black Eyed Susan blossoms. "To say I'm frustrated puts it mildly," reports homeowner, Laura Koppenhoefer. "However, if munching on this variety of plant keeps him/her away from the sunflower crop, I guess I'll just deal with it. Some of the sunflowers in a penned up area are over two and a half feet tall now!" Koppenhoefer is concerned that the local critters are developing expensive taste. "On my last trip out, I was getting tired of walking, so I didn't spend any time comparing bird food before my purchase. It turns out that I bought some sort of deluxe bird food -- it has cashews in it, for heaven's sake!" The robins, sparrows, wrens, cardinals, humming birds, black birds, black squirrels, grey squirrels, rabbits, and chipmunks all smiled, and refused request for comment.

Alone and alive
Posted Jun 27, 2012 10:18 a.m.

Some thoughts rumble around in my head. Then they go away. Others keep coming back. The ones that come back usually are ones that need something done with them and carry some thread of truth. Today's thoughts are those.

There are things that I don't really know, and perhaps can't really know, until I am alone. Alone with some thing, some one, or myself.

Alone with nature, I learn who sings for whom. I learn where the good hiding places are. I learn what uses water and when. I learn about the creativity of the Creator. I learn about renewal and things like "beginnings and endings."

Alone with my children, I learn their troubles and hopes. I learn what they remember from times I can't remember. I learn what they wrestle with. I learn what brings them joy.

Alone with my friends, I learn the ways of laughter from grown-up reflections on childhood memories. I learn the importance of sharing burdens. I learn how many people bringing together little offerings results in more than enough.

Alone with my self....I am still learning. Alone with myself in these last seven and a half years of widowhood I have known something about loneliness. I found in those years of Friday and Saturday nights that I didn't want to be alone. And was lonely, much -- especially the first three years or so, unless I was busying myself with worry for my children.

Pastors and widows know something about that lonely. I was both.

This last weekend I was alone with myself again and there was something new. I realized that not wanting to be alone was no longer the issue. I realized that, more importantly, I wanted to be alive. And I was. The gift of being alive is so much greater than being alone or together. While I am not thankful for sarcoma, I am thankful for the things I have learned with the Spirit's help, since I knew of my sarcoma. In truth, I am never truly alone. I have known this, but still had felt lonely. Certainly this shift in my priorities and awarenesses is profound for me. I am content. I have remembered and recited over and over, *Be content with such things as you have, for God God's self has said, "I will never leave you or forsake you"* (Hebrews 13:5). I certainly felt that way about my stuff, my call and my roles in life. However, in my alone time, my lonely time, I hadn't felt content for a long time. Now, I am.

I can't say that I'm glad that it took sarcoma to get over this hump. However, I am thankful that I am.

151

Learning stuff along the way; Part 2

Posted Jun 28, 2012 10:13 a.m.

There are many ways to learn things...these are just a few that capture my thoughts today:

1) Word of mouth: this is likely how Jairus, the leader of the synagogue, as well as the woman who had been hemorrhaging for twelve years learned about Jesus and his ability to heal. (Mark 5)

2) Internet: While doing a routine crop inspection yesterday, I found dozens of short horizontal rows of 1/8" holes in the ornamental pear tree in my yard. That tree had been damaged by having that huge hackberry tree land on part of it early in the spring. Via the internet, I learned that the damage is likely caused by yellow-bellied sapsuckers (a kind of wood pecker) who feast on damaged or stressed trees. I'm still hunting for how to care for my tree.

3) Demonstration: While I was visiting with my brother Eric and sister-in-law Katherine in Mississippi, Katherine picked beautiful stems of blue and purple hydrangea. She took each cut stem and dipped them in alum before putting them in the water. Weeks later, I still have over 50% of that bouquet.

4) Experience: As an elementary-aged girl, I used to love to go to the farm of my Great Aunt Lucy and Great Uncle Ray, who farmed about equal distance outside of Pontiac from us, on the opposite side of town. Their daughter Kathi was my same age. One summer Kathi and I got permission to convert a small kwansit hut (or quonset hut) that had been a chicken house into a play house for the two of us. It was like a dream come true. I don't remember a lot of the process but I do remember this: if you don't want the old chicken dookie to show, painting over it won't do it. And, just because you love the 1970s aqua-boat-dock-color paint that they gave us to use (left over from a previous project), it doesn't mean that there will be enough to cover the entire inside of the hut. Always figure the area and make sure you have enough paint for the whole project. In comparison to that first painting project, the rest of my home renovations make me look like Picasso, however, I don't think any renovations since then have been quite that fun.

5) Connections: Not "business connections," but the connectedness of family is important. After those growing up years with Lucy, Ray, Kathi and her older siblings, I haven't seen them much. My mom has stayed in contact, especially in these recent years. Last fall, my Uncle Ray died, but I wasn't well enough to be with the family for his services. This last week my Aunt Lucy died. Tomorrow I'll drive to Pontiac for the first time on my own in nine months, returning the next day, in order to connect with my family....remember with them, pray with them, laugh and cry with them. Lucy and Ray are already learning first hand of the incredible love of our incredible God.

Life and joy
Posted Jun 30, 2012 6:52 p.m.

I have a heightened awareness of little bits of healing that have really helped me reclaim some of the simple joys of living. Here are a few:
1) Some things fall in the "I-don't-take-this-for-granted-any-more" category.....for example, being able to drive over two hours by myself. I can chew mint-flavored gum now (all mint stuff was very yucky while I was on chemo). I have also had Diet Pepsi two times...not that I need to drink Diet Pepsi, but diet pop, or any cola, tasted horrible while I was on chemo.
2) Tolerating the heat. Granted, this week has been too hot for about everyone, but I am thankful to have been able to go to thirty minutes of the softball game that Sarah coached, which was wonderful to see. On chemo, I could hardly stand to be outside on a hot day.
3) Joy in listening to a concert band. For several years I played flute and piccolo with the Pontiac Municipal Band. Last night I went to their Friday evening concert -- they played beautifully -- with many songs familiar to me. The experience included the fun of greeting several high school classmates.
4) A quick recovery from a fall. While it may seem odd to be thankful for falling on the stairs, I am. On Thursday afternoon, I was carrying a small basket of laundry down the basement steps and missed the last two steps. Yeah, not so great. However, after an assessment of my assembled parts, it seemed I only twisted an ankle and "tested" the range of motion of my

right hip. After 48 hours I'm almost all better, with only a little left over ankle soreness. During the time I was on chemo, I was almost fearful of every step, and certainly afraid of every illness. My healing power was so reduced. It is a joy to move beyond feeling so very fragile.

Holding on, but not too tight
Posted Jul 5, 2012 10:49 a.m.

In these last several days I have been working on my crocheting. Yep, I admit it, I am "hooked." I've moved on to the poncho project for the two nieces. On this project, it is all about the tension. It is a soft yarn, and I am using a "K" hook, which is sort of big and makes loose stitches. I don't quite have the hang of it, but I am practicing. It would be easier if the hook was smaller and the design was tighter. But, it isn't. It is sort of like having all the control in the world over the project, but none at all.

This week in Mark 6, Jesus, who is usually on his "A-game" happens to be in his home town, where nothing seems to be working right. People think he is a bit big for his britches. He does a little healing, but that's it. Then he sends his disciples out two by two, with little instruction and fewer supplies. To me it seems a bit like telling someone to tie their shoes with one hand behind their back. I get it though, it isn't about control, it is about trust. Trusting God. Trusting that there will be people out there who will partner with you in ministry. Trusting that those people will see that they are needed in this beautiful landscape --- not just as admirers, but as workers. There is a certain "uncertainty" with the loss of control, however, there is a certain beauty when people work together, when the creative "tension" is just right, when needs are met, when a pattern forms. Thanks be to God.

Transplanted
Posted Jul 6, 2012 11:32 p.m.

The yard is going through its summer growing cycle. The coreopsis has succumbed to some mildew. The new dahlias this year are either gone (eaten by the Furry Avenger), wimpy, or thriving and blooming. The sunflowers are huge! Many are over four and a half feet tall now. Tonight, I decided that a few of them needed to try life "outside" the playpen. It was too crowded in there. I was just going to transplant two of them, but a third came up with the roots of another. I dug three holes, filled them with water that was "improved" with root stimulator, planted them, and watered some more. Tomorrow morning I'll know if they made it through the transplant.

I did my best to make the transplant go well. I minimized the time the plant was out of the ground. I dug bigger holes than were needed to get it ready to grow in ground the best. I waited until after the heat of the day to work. The very act of transplanting was a prayer of hope.

I think, though, that the key to success in the transplant process is having good, nurtured, well-preserved roots.

I think the same is true for me. For you. For us all. Good roots in family. Good roots in faith. Good roots in education. All help us grow where ever we are transplanted. That is what I am praying about these days....looking at where I am being encouraged to grow right now. Who needs encouragement? Who is encouraging me? What do I see, who do I see, when I practice "being here now?"

What I figured out...
Posted Jul 12, 2012 11:10 a.m.

So, I've looked at what I have been doing that brings me joy. Spending time in my garden "puttering." Spending time with my daughters, family, and friends. Going through 50 years of pictures (emphasis on the last 24 especially) and sorting them, in preparation for scanning some of them (I don't look forward to the scanning with joy, however). Worshipping. Healing.

When I compare that list with my list, oh say 1-8 years ago, the main thing that is missing is preaching. Now that I am beginning to feel better and my mind can focus beyond the next meal, I find that I am sinking my thoughts into preaching resources. I read blogs. I listen to commentary podcasts while I do dishes. I read the texts and "carry them around with me" for the week. However, I'm not going the same places I used to go. I'm not at someone's bedside in the hospital. I'm not planning worship. I'm not sitting with the council or some ministry team.

I guess the way that I "am" with people most closely is in prayer. So, for the past bit of time I have taken this week's text with me "to" those folks in prayer. You can try it too if you want. The Gospel reading is Mark 6:14-29 -- I can say for sure that I prayed that none of us are beheaded, like John the Baptist was!

Just below the surface
Posted Jul 13, 2012 9:44 a.m.

When the phone rings at 3:30 p.m. yesterday, Erica retrieves me from a crop survey, saying, "It's Iowa City on the phone." I take the phone and learn that it is Dr. Buckwalter's office wanting to schedule both a follow-up MRI on my hip and an office visit for me on the day that I go back to Iowa City to have another follow up CT scan of my chest and abdomen and a visit with Dr. Mo (August 21). With that reminder, I remember that I still carry around a little bit of fear just below the surface.

Then I sit on the deck swing, hoping for rain beyond the "five drops and occasional thunder" of the morning The hummingbird revisits the flower pots for the third time in ten minutes. The squirrels chase one another. And the cardinal chirps at the squirrels when they take her perch on the bird feeder. I go back to read Ephesians 1:3-14 and see that God *has blessed us in Christ with every spiritual blessing in the heavenly places.* Even right here, just below the surface.

Simple things to do to "be healed"
Posted Jul 16, 2012 10:31 a.m.

I am "on" a list serve for people with rare cancers, sarcoma being a type of rare cancer (or for people who care for those who have rare cancers).

Each day I get between one and ten research reports in my inbox. Sometimes the studies are quite a bit beyond my immediate application or interest (e.g., A phase I study of E7080, a multitargeted tyrosine kinase inhibitor, in patients with advanced solid tumors). Sometimes they are pretty "down to earth" for cancer patients (e.g., "How to Talk to Your Doctor About What You Found on the Internet").

I know that the folks who do that research, as well as the folks reading some of it (like myself) have keen interests in, you guessed it: cure.
Although I have about a ba-zillion meds at home now it seems, however none of them are "curative." Many of them help me heal one thing or another (e.g., mouth sores, stomach inflamation).

In the Gospel for this coming Sunday (Mark 6:30-34, 53-56), we hear about Jesus' ministry of healing (among other ministries). That word that he can heal people is one that resonates with the deep need of the people of that region and beyond. People are carrying their ill out into the common market place so they can be there when Jesus comes through and then, do something *so* simple......just touch the fringe of his cloak....and they would be healed. And, they were.

I really don't know what is out there that can cure me. I don't think anyone else knows the answer to this question either. I wish we did.
However, I think there are many things that can heal me. I try to keep some of these things in "front of my eyes" so that I remember to do them.

I list them here (a beginning list anyway) for me to remember, for me to encourage myself to do the simplest things, for they truly make a difference....

1) Keep drinking lots of water.
2) Keep worshiping and receiving communion.
3) Eat fruits and vegetables. Just because I didn't used to buy many fruits and vegetables, doesn't mean I have to keep that old pattern.
4) Go outside.
5) Take pictures of beautiful things in nature, like seven-foot tall sunflowers....look at them....grow those things, care for them.
6) Keep scripture in front of me, on my lips, in my heart, every day.
7) Love my family and friends.

157

8) Find a way to stay in community and do that.

9) Pray.

10) Keep moving. Do the physical therapy exercises. Find what jobs I can do in the house and outside and do them....even if I am very very sore at bedtime, it will get better, and I will get stronger.

11) Pray for others.

12) Be thankful, and give what I have to give.

I can do this. We can do this healing on the journey.

I wanna go back...

Posted Jul 20, 2012 9:34 a.m.

This week over 35,000 Lutheran Youth and their adult leaders have been learning, serving, worshiping and playing in New Orleans -- the Citizens with the Saints, from Ephesians 2, actually the Old Testament text for this coming Sunday. There was a period of time earlier this week when I thought "I wanna go back" to New Orleans, as I was at the Triennial Gathering three years ago there as well. But that is ok. They have a new thing to learn now. Even three more years later, there is still substantial healing to do in New Orleans. I can imagine they "wanna go back" to before August 29, 2005 when hurricane Katrina claimed so many lives and livelihoods. Wouldn't they want to go back and correct the engineering that created the worst civil engineering disaster in the history of the United States?

Today is Rod's and my 27th wedding anniversary. There's a part of me that wants to go back to sometime in those first nineteen years. I much rather liked celebrating our marriage with him here.

But I don't always want to go back. In fact, that whole notion is sort of a mixed bag. Last evening as the younger residents of our home were bickering over cleaning or not cleaning, I got to thinking that they didn't do that so much when I was going through surgeries and chemotherapy. Or, if they did, I didn't hear it. Now, at times, they are back at it. However, I don't want to go back. Like any parent might say, I don't want my illness to be the reason that my kids get along. I think getting along is its own motivation and reward. However, I'm only the mother. I could be wrong. In the mean time, I changed my mind. I'll stick with being here now.

Just who is Jesus, anyway?
Posted Jul 24, 2012 12:45 p.m.

It isn't noon yet and the better part of the morning was spent going to and from, and being in the doctor's office. A simple cold has become a sinus infection and bronchitis (but not pneumonia). Some time before 3:00 p.m. I will make the trip across town to the office again, after they let me know that a vial of Lidocaine (a local anesthetic) has been delivered. (I guess it is in short supply locally, and nationally.) That "numb-it" medicine will be mixed with a big-ol-dose of antibiotic in an injection into my "good hip." Then I'll start on another antibiotic, taken daily by mouth. Good. Let's get on with the healing…Healing. That's what I'm hungry for.

I took that notion to the Gospel for Sunday -- John 6:1-21. That's John's version of the feeding of the 5,000 and Jesus walking on water. Now if I was one of the hungry ones that day, or one of the disciples who got out of making a run to HyVee or to Subway to pick up 5,000 Value Meals, I would have been so thankful. If I was one of the disciples, fearfully rowing our boat on stormy seas, only to see Jesus walking on the water toward us, I'm not sure I would have been thankful, so much as freaked out. Who is He anyway? I mean, really. He certainly was a miracle worker. But it wasn't clear yet to them that He was the Son of God.

It seems that each day I read some scripture, but I also go and "read" my garden. Many days I read my garden more closely than scripture. However I think I'm looking for the same thing..or person....or, actually God, that the disciples were. Something in me wants to look at each leaf, each blossom. The closer I look, the more beauty I see in it, which is a joy in and of itself. However, the closer I look, the more beauty and wonder I have in God. I know that it isn't just doctors in their offices who have intricate knowledge of the inner workings of things. God knows. The same God who made sure people had food on the hillside and who wasn't afraid to get the hem of a robe wet to reach the frightened disciples, knows how these flowers do what they do, and how they look how they look.

The closer I look, the more I trust. The closer I look, the more I know that that one who created the beauty also created me. The closer I look, the more I know about love. The closer I look, the more I know enough about Jesus to know he is more than enough for me. I am so thankful those beautiful but ordinary flowers are a part of God's extraordinary language of love for me.

A short trip
Posted Jul 25, 2012 8:47 p.m.

Somehow it felt like the healing I had done in eight weeks was sucked right back up when I was in that spot between my cold and the bronchitis/sinus infection that was diagnosed yesterday. Because the improvement was so gradual, I had sort of (thankfully) forgotten how really lousy it is to feel really lousy. Yesterday, with the help of an injected and an oral antibiotic I am back on track -- not necessarily feeling better yet, but I can see it from where I sit.

Tonight, I remembered the fear of such times as I visited the CaringBridge site of little boy (age five or six) named Ryan, and read a post from his mom. Ryan's story is quite lengthy and I came to know it only through the site. Someone who visits my site, asked if I would hold Ryan and his family in prayer. I have, and continue to do so, along with his family. You, helping me, helped me to help them.

Just what we needed...
Posted Jul 30, 2012 11:34 a.m.

This coming Sunday, we hear again the story of those whiny, hungry, complaining Israelites in the wilderness (Exodus 16). The Lord heard their complaint and sent food....quail at night and manna in the mornings. It was just what they needed.

This last week I made a trip to my local practitioner on the advice of Dr. Mo. A routine cold had turned into a sinus infection and bronchitis. After 48 hours or so, the girls and I were headed to the Ozarks to vacation with my folks and dear family and friends at Breezy Point Resort. My family has been vacationing there since the mid-70s. As much as I really needed those antibiotics and the inhaler, I think I needed that trip to the Ozarks just as much. In as much as one can be fed by beauty and healed by immersion in love, I am so much more well now than I was five days ago.

Despite the drought, the beauty of the lake and the familiar scenes brought such joy! The opportunity to visit with lifelong friends as the sun rose and set, or while bobbing in the waves of the lake brought reminders of years of love and fun. An evening swim in the cool lake water with my mom and daughters surely must have been what the doctor ordered. Recurring "photo-ops" were staged to offer evidence of four of the best days of the year....us in the water, in the boat, on the dock, and feeding fish. My cough remains, but there is no whining or complaining from me about these days....I am well fed, loved, and "watered."

We're connected, you know
Posted Aug 1, 2012 11:12 a.m.

Every day since my diagnosis last September I have taken some sort of daily assessment of my body -- what's hurt, what's healing, what's growing, what's shrinking. Likely, I did so prior to the diagnosis as well, because I lived with growing pain for at least a year before that. My trip to the physical therapist this week revealed what I had expected, my hip is finally improving -- the range of motion, the strength and such. As my hip feels better, so do I. We're connected, you know.

Last night as I watched the exaltation and joy of the U.S. Olympic women's gymnastic team, at the same time, I was waiting for one sister in Christ to go into labor, and another sister in Christ who was giving birth to three sweet boys, many months before they were supposed to come into the world. On the Sarcoma Facebook Site, one person announces that there is no more evidence of disease. Another announces that she is preparing to have a leg and half of her pelvis removed, and yet another says that the sarcoma is taking over his lungs and liver and kidneys. With them, I sing for joy and I weep. We're connected, you know.

The whole thing leaves me hungry.... It has been two and a half weeks since I feasted at God's table, in worship. My, oh my; I need that food. I need to sit with those who are rejoicing and weeping and do the same. I need the bread and wine that holds us up, and holds us together and gives us life. Come on, Sunday, get here.

"When is it preaching?"
Posted Aug 7, 2012 11:19 a.m.

I'm in a odd sort of time for the average/usual person who has a care page. Most all times (I think) these are set up by people or their family members when there is a severe illness or injury. It is an efficient way to get information out there about what is going on -- a way to prevent "misinformation" from flourishing -- and a way to receive support as well. Some times an "acute phase" lasts a few days or weeks, or even months. I have kept writing beyond the acute phase. Now, I come closer to the end of this three-month window of healing, resting, physical therapy, connecting with family and friends, worship, joy, play, prayer, baking, writing, crocheting and more. Some things I can do again. Some things I can't.

It is good to exercise the brain we each have been given. My daily work includes thinking through the lectionary scripture in light of God's love and grace, the world in need, and my life. I've done that on these pages for some time.

I've thought about the responses to what I have been writing. There have been *many* responses, some shared publicly, some privately. The type of response that has me pondering today is seeing my writing as preaching. As a preacher, that can be perceived as the best or the worst thing to say. And, like a preacher, I know that once the words leave my mouth on a Sunday morning, or once I hit "post" on this site, what they mean is then not up to me, but rather to each person who hears or reads. Many people

162

who read scripture and then publicly connect it to daily life are in fact "preachers" (e.g., people who make their living at sharing God's Good News). I know that it is not a "preacher's job alone" to do this work, it is for us all! I know as well that some times the Good News wraps itself around me or you like a warm blanket on a cold day....and other times it hits us up-side the head like a two-by-four with the feeling we have been "preached AT" (with the feeling of a reprimand!) as well as preached-to. Some of you have used (with my permission) some of my story to help illustrate something in your own preaching on Sundays. I have been sent some of the most remarkable sermons, which show me that what I lift up is only a foretaste of a full message.

I guess, whether what I write is considered preaching or not, it is what I am learning about what helps me live every day. I have figured out what diet I need to eat when I am on a particular chemotherapy. I learned how water consumption helps me feel better. I've learned of the incredible love of my parents and daughters and family and friends. And, I've learned that having a conversation with God through the scriptures and prayer every day helps me, and heals me. It heals the spots in me that don't show up on scans or offer some sort of a number when it is counted under a microscope. Those might be some of the most important spots of all.

Then and now
Posted Aug 9, 2012 8:39 a.m.

Then...the only pie I would eat was pumpkin (or chocolate pudding pie called "confetti pie" because it had multi-colored miniature marshmallows stirred into it.)
Now...I will leave my recliner, my crocheting project, and a perfectly good evening of once-in-four-years women's beach volleyball to go eat a piece of triple-berry-pie at Village Inn with my friends.
Then...everything I needed to take to college would fit in one vehicle, including my stereo and two Panasonic Thrusters (speakers the size of furniture!) and two dozen or so albums.

Now...I'm pretty sure that it will take two trips plus some to get Sarah moved into college, and her ba-zillion songs fit on her iPod and a "dock" that is about the size of a toaster.

Then...as a little girl, I never knew anyone who had cancer, and cancer wasn't something people talked about. I figured that being a survivor meant the cancer was gone.

Now...I don't know too many families who haven't had someone close to them suffer with cancer, but I also know many people who have had cancer and are still living, thriving and loving. Today, I figure I'm a survivor already. We are all survivors of something.

Then...I learned the song "Jesus Loves Me, This I Know."

Now...I'm still singing the same song.

To do one thing...
Posted Aug 10, 2012 11:02 p.m.

Last night I had an idea of what I would say today. That is sort of unusual. Usually, my idea comes in the morning. This morning, that idea was gone. I knew it was one thing. One simple thing.

My day progressed. I was a friend. I was a mom. I couldn't remember the one thing. I crocheted. I ate pizza. I wasn't remembering at all. I had another thought and called a friend to tell her something and before she said "Hello," I forgot what I was going to tell her. It was only one thing. Oh bother. I took a little longer walk to the south end of Swanie Slough on Augustana's campus (about four blocks away) and breathed in the cool green of the slough...a beauty to behold (even if I can't walk the height/length of the slough yet). I ironed my clothes to wear to a family cook-out tomorrow. I cheered on the Olympians.

Then I remembered. Last night before I went to bed I had checked the Sarcoma Alliance site on Facebook. Someone was ready to give up on chemo because the nausea was so so bad. I've not only visited that "location" in life, it was my address for a few days. I offered my suggestions, adding to the encouragements and prayers of many others who have walked that path. I thought, "well....if I could only do one thing today, this was enough to do...to reach out, as people had reached out to me."

Healing by being me
Posted Aug 13, 2012 9:45 a.m.

Today is a recovery day, and that is all right. Yesterday, I was able to preach and preside at St. John's Lutheran Church in Rock Island for my friend, Stacie Fidlar, as she enjoyed some vacation time. The timing of it all was a blessing to me. At two weeks out from scan-time, I was beginning to experience "scanxiety." So, the meditation on the texts for the week, the focus of preparation to preside in a new place, the joy of doing familiar things such as text study and of using much loved resources .....well, it was just what Dr. Mo would have ordered.

With Stacie's help (as well as the help of some great parishioners) we adapted a few things so I could conserve energy....for instance, I didn't do the communion distribution myself and I sat on a stool to offer greetings at the end of worship. I was also blessed to have a whole row of worshiping-cheerleading-encouraging people at worship. It seems that in the fight to kick this cancer out, I am also encouraged along the way by remembering who I am and how I am called to serve.

This week I prepare for two events in three days......the "taking of the daughter Sarah to college" and the "day-o-scans" in Iowa City (on Sunday and the following Tuesday, respectively). I think that my preparation will call for embracing each day for the blessing it is, drinking lots of water, prayer, reading, laundry, writing, physical therapy exercises, and, with any luck, chocolate.

Reframing the calendar
Posted Aug 15, 2012 10:35 a.m.

The other day I was going through the cedar chest in the dining room for table linens. I found those, and also came across the First Year Calendars that I kept for the girls. First smiles. First cheerios. First time climbing on top of the sofa/counter/table. Baptism. First tooth. First time throwing her toys in the toilet (her, not me). I kept one year of calendaring for Erica and two years for Sarah (because we didn't video tape as much of Sarah).

Yesterday, when I didn't write here, it was because I was having a big "calendar day." We were investigating what we thought was Sarah's first broken bone (in her foot) which turned out not to be broken, but is in need of wearing the shoe portion of one of those "boots" for three weeks anyway. (This is oh so handy as she is in the midst of packing to return to college on Sunday).

Erica started a new type of job at Target and a second job, as a nanny and planning a bridal shower for her best friend.

So far, thinking about the calendar in these sorts of ways is more distracting than thinking about using it to count down to scans. Any time I can do it, it is better to count blessings than troubles.

Not worth it versus worth it
Posted Aug 17, 2012 9:29 a.m.

Not worth it: Trying a "no pain med day" because by 3:00 p.m. my choices were either (1) cry in the recliner, or (2) take something for the aching.

Asking for all the dirty dishes from upstairs...because they never ALL arrive at once. I think they reproduce somehow.

Taking my camera outside to try to capture the beauty of one of the yellow finches feeding on the sunflower seeds. (It is easier to capture images of the hummingbirds!)

Worth it: Making big family lunches two days in a row to be able to have my two daughters with me, telling stories and just having fun together.

Having a project to work on that takes a lot of concentration (like reconciling all of my receipts on Quicken).

Asking for prayers for peace as I wait for the scans.

Going to physical therapy as the exercises really seem to be helping the hip.

Learning new technologies, because I love Skyping with family and friends who live too far away for me to see regularly.

Keeping the kitchen really clean and picked up, because people (including me) are less likely to leave dirty dishes just sitting around.

Accepting help with the lawn care this summer. Even though there hasn't been very much mowing needed, the mulching, weeding, trimming, blowing, and "removal of dead squirrel parts from the shed" are so very much appreciated.

Regular worship, because I am hungry for more than just chocolate.

Reading the Gospel texts from John these last many weeks....it is bread which is talked of over and over....which is like God saying "I love you, I love you, I love you" over and over.

Collecting boxes, because Sarah can use them to pack to go to college in two more days....back to school is a bittersweet time....but worth it in the long term.

Good reasons to "scan"
Posted Aug 18, 2012 10:21 p.m.

Reason #1:
Scanning-in pictures from the 50 years of sorting has begun. I started with the brand-new-baby pictures of Sarah. They are so wonderful. With my new phone upgrade, those same pictures are now on both computers and my phone. There's a lot of love and joy to carry around in something the size of a deck of cards....and in my heart too.....right at the time when part of my heart goes back to college for her sophomore year at Illinois State.

<u>Reason #2:</u>
A year ago this "time" as Sarah was moved-in to college, my mom "scanned" my pain-filled-walking and saw that my right hip was swollen. She asked "Did I know that?" Not really, it just hurt. I'm glad Mom scanned me.

<u>Reason #3:</u>
Smart, well trained people scan parts of my "insides" and then, based on those scans, they can figure out how to get me better.

<u>Reason #4:</u>
I've scanned that Bible again...the theme still seems to be "I love you, forever" and "Love one another." These are good things to remember in light of 1, 2, 3 and the like.

Intersecting stories
Posted Aug 20, 2012 10:45 p.m.

In any good story you hear of one person whose life impacts another, who influences another. It doesn't just happen in stories, it happens in life. Every day. In the best possible ways and in the most sorrowful ways, it happens.

Yesterday, I took Sarah to Illinois State to start her sophomore year...it was a wonderful day. Heading back to "Normal," literally is like going home for Sarah. That is where she was born. Many members of her family (including one grandmother and grandfather) are ISU Alumni.

Sometime last night, my mother-in-law, Dorothy Elaine Koppenhoefer suffered a stroke. The effect of it seems more pronounced this evening than it was this morning. While she receives loving care at Meadows Mennonite Home in their Alzheimer's unit, it is difficult for those of us in her family to be apart from her during this struggle. On behalf of her (our) family, we appreciate your care and prayers.

Tomorrow, my folks and I will head to Iowa City, arriving around 6:45 a.m., with scans at 7:20 and 9:30, and doctor appointments at 10:30 and 11:40. I know that however hard or closely they look "inside" at me, that they will find that some part of me is actually in Normal with Sarah, and at Meadows with Elaine.....just like the rest of her loving family.

Good news at last....
Posted Aug 21, 2012 5:11 p.m.

As someone who has preached the Good News for many years, it feels so good to actually receive some sometimes!
In short...
1) No chemo (...I had already thought about how I was going to deal with losing my hair).
2) The lung tumors and pleural effusions (pockets of fluid in the bases of each lung) are only slightly larger...not larger-enough to start to attack with chemo.
3) My liver is all back to normal.
4) The tissue in my hip looks great according the scan assessment of Dr. Buckwalter....it is hard to even tell which hip had the surgery!
5) The achy feeling that I continue to have, especially in my joints is not related to the cancer (big relief there), rather it is because of the chemo -- which had a sort of "rapid aging effect" on my joints.
6) The lump on top of my ankle is likely a nerve ganglion (and not cancer)....however, after a few moments of assessment, one doctor just about got kicked!
7) The shoulder pain is going to be addressed by physical therapy..all the doctors quickly dismiss me as being a surgical candidate.
8) I go back for rescanning in 3 months again.... AND
9) Dr. Mo is quite hopeful that this slow rate of growth will be the norm... I would like "No growth" but I'll take slow.....maybe even for a year!
And....my mother-in-law is going to the hospital for some tests. Her doctor wants to make sure there isn't something fixable going on and not a stroke.
Rest. Breathe. Hope.

"...this teaching is hard...."
Posted Aug 25, 2012 9:52 p.m.
The gospel this week comes from John 6....here is just a bit of it. Jesus says... *58: This is the bread that came down from heaven, not like that which your ancestors ate, and they died. But the one who eats this bread*

will live forever. 59: He said these things while he was teaching in the synagogue at Capernaum. 60: When many of his disciples heard it, they said, "This teaching is difficult; who can accept it?"

This has been quite a week. I have to admit....perhaps a bit like those shocked disciples that not everything I heard on Tuesday was easy to hear. It actually helped me this week to have a few days in care of my mother-in-law to digest the words from Dr. Mo. Even in the face of so much really good news, that bit about "the tumors growing" seemed to weigh disproportionally large with me. One friend who has been in a similar position describes this as something like "life in the waiting room."

For a few days, I actually felt badly that I was not as happy as the people whom I told to be happy! As thankful as I was and am to be waiting, I sure wish I didn't have anything to wait for. Yep, this teaching is hard.

However, on Wednesday I was able to join others from Rod's family to support and encourage my mother-in-law at Advocate BroMenn Medical Center in Normal Illinois as she began some steps for recovery from a stroke. This is the hospital where I worked as a student nurse, nurse, nursing educator, and chaplaincy student....and met my husband, and gave birth to Sarah. There is a lot of wonderful history there. While I wish this wasn't a part of our history there, I am glad that this place was ready to offer her care. Elaine was in the newly opened wing of the center. It was a wonderful place to be as a family, and her care there was superb. She is a strong woman of great courage, and although the teaching she had, and will have is hard (like eating, sitting, using her right arm and hand, speaking easily), she has shown some improvements.

As a person who has been a care giver for much of my adult life, it has been hard for me to be on the receiving end for the majority of the last year. (....that teaching is hard....) However, I have very much appreciated that care. In the last three days, I got to return some of the loving care I have received, and have been part of a family-wide effort to be present for a courageous, loving woman.

Remembering at a football game

Posted Aug 31, 2012 11:09 p.m.

Last year.... I was at a Rocky football game (for the marching band, especially). I had just learned that I had a tumor in my hip, but didn't know what it was "made of" and wouldn't know that for just a few days.

This year... tonight....I was at the Rocky/Metamora football game (for the marching band, especially). In this year I've learned a zillion things...like what the tumor was made of, and what I am made of, and what my wonderful family and super friends and amazing congregation...and hope is made of. Only one of those things was horrible....the rest were good.

A few numbers

Posted Sept 6, 2012 9:29 p.m.

One cup of coffee in the morning. Just enough. Not too much.

Two remarkable stories of healing by Jesus in the Gospel for Sunday...a daughter at the pleading of a mother and a deaf man at the begging of his friends (Mark 7:24-37).

Twenty-four smiley face cake pops made by Erica for the "Cake Walk" at St. John's East End Neighborhood Fair on Saturday afternoon.

Fifty-one years will be celebrated by me in October. Currently trying to figure out how to celebrate -- and celebrate I will! And I encourage all of you to celebrate your birthdays when you have them, and you know you will! Celebrate life!

One hundred years of ministry and life in the community of Christ is being celebrated by Trinity Lutheran Church in Moline this year. It is bittersweet to have been a part of the congregation for the last eight years or so and not to be a part of this past year with them. My primary call for the last year has been healing -- a full time job that has been better because of the support and prayers of so many. However, tomorrow, with the encouragement of the synod and the invitation of the congregation, I will join them for their anniversary banquet. Life in Christ is all worth celebrating.

171

Just praying
Posted Sep 8, 2012 12:19 p.m.

I don't remember all of the details that go with the background of this story, but I am so overwhelmed with the beauty of the Spirit at work that I feel compelled to tell it.

Scene one: My bathroom mirror. I use it to post things to remind me of God's love, my daughters, encouragements, prayer reminders and the like. On the mirror is a name: Atong. She is the 16-year-old daughter of Michael who works at Trinity Lutheran. She was in the Kakuma refuge camp in Kenya. During the time I was at Trinity, I tried, as did others, through national Lutheran channels to help Michael get his daughter to the U.S. Nothing was working. During this year at home, I just prayed. I saw her name, and prayed.

Scene two: Table number five at the Centennial Celebration Banquet at the Botanical Center last night. A table mate said that she took Michael and his family to pick up Atong at the airport in the Quad Cities. What? Really? The story of travel here included the work of members of Trinity Lutheran here and in Washington, D.C., and a local politician and World Relief. I saw Atong for the first time via an iPhone as the reunion had been captured in pictures.

We were celebrating 100 years of ministry and a highlight of that ministry -- the faith in action of a few people, loved by God, loving the neighbor -- happened right there. That is it. Beyond the buildings and programs and employees and pastors (yes, even pastors)....God's work. Our hands. The story of God's love had been told and retold for over 100 more years, and tonight our thanksgivings include a family reunited.

Scene three: Nine months or more ago. I remember feeling frustrated as I felt so sick, looking at my mirror. I tried to remember and to memorize some scripture. I put it on my mirror, but I couldn't get it to stick in my head. So frustrating. I put other stuff there. I put Atong's name there. I just prayed. I knew people were praying for me too.

Scene four: Entering the Botanical Center last night...and then going into the banquet room, I was overwhelmed by seeing the faces of so many people who have been praying for me for so long. Praying for me, even though there wasn't anything else they could "do." "Just pray." I asked, and they have.

Scene five: Now. In the recliner. After ten hours of sleep, meds, breakfast and coffee. I am still incredibly grateful, and hopeful. I am thankful to have been a part of the care of Atong, and so thankful for those who helped her family finally figure out the inner workings of the maze that made it possible for her to reunite with her father and family. I am thankful for the people who want so much to do something more than "just pray" for me and my family.

We all need to know this: there is no "Just" to praying. It is not a lesser thing. It is not a thing of last resort. It is a practice of communication with the One who loves and creates us. And it is more than enough.

To sing
Posted Sep 10, 2012 11:00 a.m.

I do most of my singing in worship. Over this last year I've experienced my ability to sing almost disappear (because of shortness of breath) and reappear (as the shortness of breath subsided). Sometimes I couldn't sing because I was crying. Sometimes I would sing to keep from crying.

But sometimes, more recently, I find the singing is a statement to my lungs: "Listen to this. This is the Good News. There are a number of you lung cells that have decided not to play nicely with the others. Just because I am not clobbering you with chemotherapy does not mean that I am ok with you being there. The fact that you include sarcoma cancer cells and not typical lung cancer cells makes no difference. You are still not welcome. I have decided to kill you with kindness. I will bathe you in songs and hymns."

A person, a family, a city, a nation, the world
Posted Sep 11, 2012 10:36 a.m.

I began reading Deanna Thompson's book, *Hoping for More*, in this break that I am taking between Ken Follett's books, *Pillars of the Earth* and *World Without End*. In "Pillars," I read at the rate of about 50 pages a day for that 950-page feast. In the last two days I have been pushed to read 38 pages total of Deanna's book. It is hard to read quickly when I am sobbing. It has been quite a while since the early months of my diagnosis when I was crying for significant parts of every day. I admit that it is hard to go back to that, even if for a "re-journey" with a book that covers some similar ground for her experience of Stage IV breast cancer.

There is something in there for me though. I don't know what it is yet, but I will keep reading. One thing I have figured already is the enormity of what my physical, emotional and spiritual being has been through in the past year -- and the beauty of the grace that has been poured on me by my family, friends and so many others.

Today, on September 11, the air seems filled with story. Stories pour out of people and cities and nations. The grieving from that day continues. The striving for peace continues as well. Telling those stories is a part of healing.

Today, I imagine God encouraging us to tell, read, hear, the ongoing story of hope and healing for all God's people. In telling that story, we speak God, ever-present -- ready and willing to bear our sorrows with us, and re-create us in the ways of peace.

Why, oh, why....
Posted Sep 12, 2012 6:01 p.m.

Yesterday, I took a big step. I went back to RIFAC, the Rock Island Fitness and Activity Center. I had been a regular for the first eight years that we've lived in town. I would go twice a week for the first few years, and then three times a week for the more recent years. This last year has been different. I could have gone even a month ago or more, but I didn't. Or, couldn't....

I don't think I am the only one who wrestles with going or not going to the gym.

For as many times as I have thought someone (besides me) should go to the gym, or told them to go to the gym, I am sorry for that many times. Ok, maybe not. However, I do see that trip differently now.

RIFAC had been the place I went to walk or lift weights, play racquetball or swim. It revived my spirit as much as it did my body. I met wonderful people in my community, and years ago, as a grieving wife and mother, just the act of getting out of the house for something other than work or groceries was a herculean feat.

It is a place where I grew strong and hopeful. It is the place where I could tell that I was healing after surgeries. It is the place where I walked and meditated on the scriptures, writing more sermons than I could begin to count. Through the windows, I watched seasons come and go -- admiring the beauty of them all.

Then I couldn't go back.

That was the place where the body that I trusted tried to tell me something was wrong. At least three years before my diagnosis, I had pain in my hip when I played racquetball. In the months before my diagnosis the pain was so severe that I would be pulled up short when I walked. Within a matter of a few scans and some highly educated eyes, my RIFAC days came to an abrupt halt.

I had wanted, even planned to return to RIFAC at the first of the year. Chemotherapy and the need to stay away from "germ exposure" plus the inability to drive, and shortness of breath were among the reasons I stayed away. Walking from the parking lot, uphill, to the front door was the outer limit of my capacity to "hike."

I can walk now though. I can even get on the stationary bike. But why couldn't I go?

After I got there, I thought that through....and realized I had been afraid that I would cry my way around that track. The new me missed the old me -- the one that felt confident, and healthy, and sure that there were countless years and opportunities ahead. It is hard to work out in front of others when I am so busy trying to work things out in my head. How is it that I can look so much better and even feel better and still be carrying stage 4 cancer around in my body? There is so much more to being better than looking better. I want the whole package.

I don't have answers to these things yet, and likely will be wrestling with them for some time to come. However, some things were made much better by being at RIFAC. I tried some of the things I used to do.....listen to podcasts, listen to music and look for the beauty of nature in the surrounding area.

I will go back to RIFAC. I wrestle with not being able to go back in time. I'm not the only one who has had that thought either. It is important to make myself as healthy as I can be. I'm not the only one who has had that thought either. When I go back, I'll be praying for me and all those of us who have many reasons why it is hard to take the first step, again.

Reading, remembering, celebrating
Posted Sep 15, 2012 10:59 a.m.

Reading....done with Deanna Thompson's book, *Hoping for More*. Despite the crying that ensued, I highly recommend this book...especially for people who have/have had cancer, and the people who love them. Her experiences with the blessings of the community that is made via Caring Bridge (in her case) and CarePages (in my case) she calls "the Virtual Body of Christ" --- her experience of the church universal. It is a remarkable thing and I am deeply grateful as well. She spends some time reflecting on and responding to people's comments about her cancer, as well as theodicy (a fancy word for God's role--or not--in human suffering and human sinfulness). Remembering.....Rod's Aunt Sylvia Jacobsen, who passed away in July and was remembered yesterday in her memorial service and family luncheon in Joliet. It was a good day to spend with Rod's extended family, who are also CarePage readers, and good "huggers" and lifted my spirits with "You look great" comments through the day.
Celebrating....my dad's birthday (with the gift of a book he has already read....rats....will try again on that front) and my mother-in-law Elaine's 90th birthday tomorrow with a gathering of family. (I come bearing anise springerle and lime-coconut springerles for the gathering.)
And, I celebrated Family Weekend at Illinois State with Sarah, by spending time with her today after her work at the Children's Discovery Museum and will tomorrow with Community of Joy worship at St. John's Lutheran in Bloomington.
This has been a good week and weekend to practice "Be here now." I am so very blessed. Right here right now is a wonderful place to be.

One Year
Posted Sep 27, 2012 10:51 a.m.

I knew this day was coming. I couldn't remember the "date." I've gotten so dependent on that little number (27) to show up on the dock of my MacBook Pro, or on the opening page of my iPhone. Yep that's it. On September 27, 2011, Mom, Dad, and I went to Iowa City. I had the scans. I went from doctor to doctor. The news was worse each time.

A number of times over the last year I wrote posts entitled "things that help" -- I've also written posts that included what I was thankful for. Those things still stand.

Today, I give thanks for the Word....The Living Word of Christ present with us, the preached Word, and the written Word. As I have struggled over this past year, it has been the Word in these three ways that has kept me from despair (or at least from making despair my permanent address). Psalm 19:14 *Let the words of my mouth and the meditation of my heart be acceptable to you, O Lord, my rock and my redeemer.*
One year. Still here.

The "To Do" List
Posted Sep 28, 2012 11:31 a.m.

Where do you keep your "to do" list? A good portion of my list is in a frog's-head-shaped-spiral-note-pad. I like to make lists and check things off when they are done. I do best when my list is somewhere that I can see it. If I can't see it, it may not be there to do. Right? When the list is found again --whoa I am surprised by all there is to do! (Perhaps this is the adult's version of Peek-a-Boo.) However, perhaps the best place to put a to-do list is on the refrigerator. I never lose my refrigerator.

Lately my ongoing list has physical therapy and exercise on it. I have now added swimming to that list of exercises I can do. Thirty minutes in the pool this week seems to have done more good than harm, so I am likely to return. I have an ongoing "to-do" list for my yard, as the deck and fence are going to be rebuilt. The demolition work started today. Actually, I shouldn't say that. The demolition work has been going on for years due to some wood rot, and some hungry termites. Thankfully the house has no termites. As the girls have said, "let's just feed them more fence."

Some things are on hold, like laundry. The washer no longer has any spinning action whatsoever. We are in day two of a seven-day wait for the repair person to get to us on their list.

To top off my "to do" list, I have figured out the ten-step process for finding my lost (or stolen?) driver's license:
1) look for a week.
2) call the high school where you think you lost it.
3) search through the home-side press box in the football stadium in case someone turned it in there.
4) search the stands (three days after it is lost).
5) empty out your purse/billfold 10-12 times.
6) search your bedroom and linens 2-3 times.
7) look under your bed many times but do not put
"vacuum under bed" on the list of things to do so that there is not a dust-allergy-induced sneezing fit each time I look.
8) go to the Department of Motor Vehicles to get a new license (call non-emergency police number to make sure I do not need a police report number in order to get a new license; search the DMV web-site to see what I need to bring along; call the local DMV to make sure the on-line list is correct; have eldest daughter drive me to DMV because the thought of having an accident or problem with no license on me sends me into a financial fit; spend 23 minutes there and 23 minutes driving each direction from/to the DMV; be waited on by three DMV employees; write a check for $5; go home with my new duplicate license.
9) two days later ask elder daughter to vacuum out the Highlander.
10) she finds license in-between the front seats. Done. Check finding license off to-do list. Figure out what to do with two licenses. (Imagine the "street market" value of a 50-year-old-white-female license for those who

want to get on AARP but are not quite old enough. Rule out all strategies that have the words "street market" in them and shred original license.)

Here is a reminder of something for all of us to do....as a part of my virtual 51st birthday celebration (a week from today-- October 5th)--You can even post this on your refrigerator:
Buy peanut butter or tuna.
Donate it to your local food bank/food pantry.
Smile. (Think, "Hurray! Happy Birthday, Laura! Happy eating to somebody's family!")
Thankful that all our pictures are on God's refrigerator.

A fine line...
Posted Oct 2, 2012 5:09 p.m.

I remember the feeling that I had seven years or so ago as I emerged from a grief-filled fog after Rod's death. I certainly wasn't invincible, but I felt like I had a remarkable amount of courage. "What could you do to hurt me now?! Nothing!" When I held whatever challenging experience I had in the light of day, I felt like nothing could be worse than the loss of my husband (with the exception of if something happened to my daughters). Car troubles or a messy house or work challenges or whatever could never rate much higher than a 3 or 4 when I had experienced a 10.

I've talked to veterans who describe something similar upon returning from war. Everything is great in comparison to what they experienced.

The thing is, that feeling doesn't last forever. Whether the experience was something drawn from the well of mountain tops or deepest valleys, the road levels back out once again.

Well, of course, I found out what most of us find out. New lousy stuff does happen. And, the 9s and 10s we think could never come back, do.

I feel like I am in some new, uncharted personal territory now though. When my pain was intractable or when the effects of chemotherapy flattened me out or put me back in the hospital, I felt like my emotional and physical state matched my diagnosis and prognosis. Now, I'm feeling so much better physically than I was but experience emotional wrestling

179

that can take me to the mat because of the disparity between my physical state and what is happening inside that is visible only to God and to trained physicians at three month intervals.

To make it best from day to day, I pray, I use distraction....and I also allow myself to "forget" what is going on when I can. That said, the effect of going through this cancer journey has me wanting to keep the "re-ordering of priorities" that dealing effectively with cancer can provide me. Here is the odd thing; in order to get that "big benefit," I have to remember (at some level) that I have stage 4 cancer. That is a fine fine line to walk. Forget.....remember.....forget.....remember.

Courage
Posted Oct 8, 2012 11:18 a.m.

Courage doesn't happen in a vacuum. In the last few days I have been surrounded by the prayers and encouragements and joy of friends and family via the internet, cards, and in person...all celebrating my 51st birthday....and a year of living with and beyond my cancer.

At my folks house on Saturday, it was my honor to introduce to one another; the family and friends that had gathered there, several of whom had never met one another, or if they had met, it was for our wedding, 28 years ago. I surveyed the room. Every one of them has been a part of my healing and hope....and represent the countless others who have done the same. That circle of folks brought to mind a "trust exercise" that I have led or participated in at confirmation camps. The participants stand together in a very tight six foot diameter circle. One participant stands in the center with his/her arms crossed over his/her chest, and closes his/her eyes. Then the person (holding themselves tall and rigid) falls back into the palms of the people behind them, and then is passed forward and back, side to side, held upright by the attentive and caring group that surrounds.I know that a group is there for me and my family. I know that group is a gift from God. I also know that any courage that is required of me from day to day, is made possible because of God's presence in you, for us....attentive, caring, praying, encouraging support.

Joys of the day...
Posted Oct 10, 2012 3:47 p.m.

Joys of the day? Here are a few:
1) Seeing a friend at the fitness center, whom I had not seen since before my diagnosis last year.
2) writing a sermon (for real) while I walked at the fitness center.
3) Chinese food with Erica for lunch.
4) the joy in Sarah's voice as she told me about the townhouse that she and her roommates have selected for next year....of course a part of that joy came with me depositing $185 in her account for the security deposit.
5) seeing the footings poured for the deck and the slats go on the new fence, and knowing there are no termites in either.
6) preparing to celebrate my Erica's 24th birthday tomorrow.
7) learning to knit (in the round) fingerless, cable-backed wool mittens for Erica.
8) the sunshine of a beautiful day.
9) a bouquet of zinnias from my garden.
10) enough peace, patience, and hope for this day.

In the quiet afternoon
Posted Oct 13, 2012 3:27 p.m.

In the quiet afternoon
rooms echo stories told
of carving pumpkins years ago.

In the quiet afternoon
those orange globes
warmed from tea lights
cast shadows
away from a grey sky.

In the quiet afternoon
the house
and I
breathe and sigh
and long for the next time
the three of us gather 'round
the table smiling, laughing, carving pictures, making secrets, telling tales.

In the quiet afternoon
love and
memories stack
like treasures
heaped up
spilling over
filling up
this quiet afternoon.

Broken and open...
Posted Oct 16, 2012 11:01 a.m.

Today is "port-flushing" day. The folks at the infusion center at Trinity Hospital on 7th Street in Moline are so very kind. My "port-flushing" has gone well each time. I expect the same today. Of course, this means that in a month I will be back in Iowa City for scans and doctor visits. Somehow these two months have passed pretty quickly. In as much as I "work" to keep my port open, so that it is ready for use if needed, I have been pondering what else I am open to and what else I am learning at this stage in my living/healing/striving.

In the past few months I have been open to the Spirit's calling to serve in some small ways in ministry -- beyond my praying and writing and call-in-daily-life. I was able, with the help of a dear friend who did the driving, to preach and preside for the morning worship services for the people of God at Grace Lutheran in Knoxville on this past Sunday. I enjoyed the preparation and the day. However, I will pray long and hard about serving for a two-service Sunday.....I had a pretty long recovery phase. I don't mind being tired, but I'm not a big fan of pain. Again, I chose to do this...I learned from it...I was able to dine with friends in Galesburg at noon....and it was "Camel Sunday"....how could I pass on it!? (refer to Mark 10:17-31 for the camel's appearance).

Starting in November, I'm going to lead a weekly class for two local churches. I don't anticipate that they will be as physically challenging for me to lead as this past Sunday's worship. The odd thing about this whole thing (at least today) is that by being open to these ministries, my physical brokenness is re-revealed. That is so odd, because in serving in these ways, I find myself striving to reclaim the ways that I am whole. Most simply: on this sunny fall day, I want serving to bring happiness, not sadness. Maybe the sadness is just an alone time experience, just a part of grieving not being able to minister with the same energy and involvement that I used to do. Perhaps I need to shift my focus.

In moments this past Sunday I found joy in so so many places:

In my friend who was smiling even though I arrived at her house in the 6:15 a.m. darkness for her to drive me an hour away for a morning of ministry.

In the welcome of the woman who greeted us at Grace, got us parking and hot coffee ready all by 7:15 a.m.

In the open hands to receive Christ's body.

In the smiles and stories of the Sunday school children and their teachers.

In telling my F.R.O.G. witness in worship, and using Gamal the camel for the child's word, and of how all things are possible with God.

In the singing of "Be Thou My Vision" and the other hymns of worship.In offering blessing on the assembly, I was blessed as well.

183

Things to do today...
Posted Oct 19, 2012 11:27 a.m.

1) Enjoy choosing a necklace for the maid of honor (Erica) to wear to the wedding rehearsal this evening.
2) Pray my thanksgivings for my daughters, family and friends.
3) Stretch....and see how much my hip has healed since surgery one year ago today to have the tumor removed.
4) Accept what I can do, and what I can't do.
5) See the movie *Frankenweenie.*
6) Knit more on the cable-patterned-fingerless-mittens for Erica (after an email conversation that spanned two days with Jen, the customer service person from the yarn shop "Purl Soho" in Soho, New York, to clarify some unclear directions for said mittens).
7) Accept that there will be tears tomorrow at Erica's friend Liz's wedding. (There are already tears today.) I am used to being the pastor. Imagining this as a mom is a whole different thing.
My prayer....to be there on these sorts of days for my daughters.

Being while becoming
Posted Oct 20, 2012 2:06 p.m.

Just for the looking
Beauty
is happening all around.

One amazing leaf
yellow and red
appeared beside my house.
So pretty it was that it caught my eye twice
and a third time I stooped
to take a picture.

One dear crocheting friend
so loving her daughter

184

picked up knitting needles and chased orange yarn around them
taming it into a tiny pattern.
Soft, deep heather yarn
waits for skill to grow
to become a gift of love that looks like a scarf.

One daughter of mine
reached out for a little conversation
only to find me immersed in helping others.
Later that night
her sweet response to my electronic apology
revealed such tenderness
as would make me all the more longing for the next time we talk.

The other daughter
stepped out of her work role
for days of celebration
as the maid of honor for her best friend.
Gowns and shoes reveal one kind of beauty...
but the beauty of
her friendship and care
understanding and shared story are breath-taking.

All I had to offer was a glance
and I was given glimpses of beauty all around.
The beauty of being while becoming.

Things that help; Part 10
Posted Oct 23, 2012 12:21 p.m.

1) I've been thinking this last week about things that help me now. This morning I came upon the Gospel for this coming Sunday: the story of Jesus' healing of blind Bartimaeus. (Mark 10:46-52) Jesus says to Bartimaeus, "Your faith has made you well." And, Bartimaeus was healed of his blindness. Faith helps. It not only helps, it heals. And by "it heals," I mean faith in the One who created, saved, and sustains us, heals. I don't

185

think I'm in a very exclusive club of folks who would, believing, like to run up to Jesus and say "Hey, a little healing here please!" In fact, I do that pretty much every day. The fact that I still have sarcoma and I still pray for healing does not diminish my faith, or Christ's effectiveness as a healer. Truly, I know through my faith that I am being healed and forgiven and sustained and challenged and blessed and encouraged every day.One area that really needed the healing was my trust in God that I would have enough financially to sustain myself and my daughters. (This worry was there, even though I have the promise of support from my family and the generous gifts of so many through the FUNdraiser last year.) I knew that the "one year review" of my disability was coming up and I was concerned that because I "look good" (so you all say) and because I feel better than I did when I was on chemotherapy that I would loose a portion or all of my disability and have to perform in a work setting beyond my physical capacity to do so.This last weekend, weeks before I thought I would know, I learned that my long-term, long term disability has been approved. This is such an incredible relief. I can still "minister" in small ways to supplement my spirit and my income, but do not have to work to the point of jeopardizing my health. The support of my family and the support of this disability is grace....all grace. And it is healing. This helps.

2) Being "one year away" (from my diagnosis and from leaving my call) helps....as does the open and honest work in grieving those losses. The pain of leaving my call was as much a physical pain as was the tumor. A year ago, the acceptance of disability felt like "failure" on my part. It isn't. This support gives me room to heal in every way possible. Perhaps there will be a day when I do not need it any more on this side of eternity.

3) Rain helps. It is good to see the lawn green again. It is good to see the zinnias still blooming. I remind myself of this, as the humidity is not so much a help on the joints in my body!

4) Looking ahead to teaching again helps. I'll be leading a class on the book, *Seven Spiritual Gifts of Waiting,* by Rev. Holly Whitcomb. One hour on a Sunday. One hour on a Wednesday. I can do this and I ask God to help and guide me.

5) Writing to Sarah.... this really helps Sarah. It is a very heavy year for her at Illinois State and she has mused that when I was in chemotherapy she got a ton of mail. She has repeated to me that she *does not* want me to

get sicker. Period. However, helping my daughter helps me too, and she loves letters.

6) Delivering the peanut butter and tuna which people donated for my birthday in lieu of a gift. I kid you not, "spreading" the love around felt amazing. I'm thinking about adding one jar of peanut butter and a can of tuna to my regular shopping, and then delivering a bag when it looks "about right." What heals me, heals others too.

7) Praying for others, helps. Like praying for those I know who are experiencing a loss, those who are awaiting a transplant or recovering from one, those who have had a stroke, those who are looking for work, those who are separated from family, those who are worrying, those who are preparing for travel, those who are newly married,....and you.

A worshipper or a tourist
Posted Oct 29, 2012 3:55 p.m.

This last Saturday, Penny invited me to join her on a trip to Valparaiso University. We were striving to get there and get checked in so that we could attend a chapel tour that started at 11 a.m. We got there and joined a tour that had just begun....finding them at the baptismal font, where Penny's daughter had been baptized just a few weeks ago. Although I had been told of the beauty of the chapel countless times, I don't think I was prepared for the impact that it would have on me. With the exquisite telling of the story and theology of the chapel itself, by the LCMS Pastor Jim and ELCA Pastor Char, I (we) were enfolded into the story of and life of Christ and the lives of all who follow Christ.

Climbing up into the pulpit reminded me of standing in Luther's pulpit in the Castle Church in Wittenberg, Germany. Walking down into the chapel under the main altar reminded me of walking down into the chapel under the main altar in the Church of the Nativity in Bethlehem. In those international two places, I was a tourist. A Christian sister....but a tourist non-the-less. But at Valpo, in the Chapel of the Resurrection, I was not a tourist. Not even on Saturday. I was a worshipper. Each time they told me something new or explained some architectural feature, in my mind I said "Amen"....Yes....It is so.

The next day, after other tours and shopping and lovely meals and meeting the daughter and friends, we were back at the chapel, for Reformation Sunday worship. Pastor Char presided and a Deaconess preached a wonderful sermon on discipleship Anyway. The point is that I never felt like a tourist. I felt a part of the Christian community that is distinctly and beautifully Lutheran....striving to be LCMS and ELCA together and beyond. We worshipped and communed together.

Across the aisle, sat Walter Wangerin, Jr., a Lutheran hero of mine. A wonderful author, teacher and presenter, who wrote more recently, *Letters from the Land of Cancer*, reflecting on his diagnosis and life with lung cancer. I forgot that he was on faculty at Valpo. And there he was. After worship I introduced myself and thanked him for writing that particular book and said that I still prayed for him on that journey. I couldn't figure much else to say....perhaps, just a bit star-struck.

Yet, star-struck or not, I left. No, I take that back. I was sent. Sent into the world to serve. All good, true, worship does that for me. Yep. I was sent, am sent, along with Walter Wangerin, Jr. and Penny and the students and the faculty and the staff and the people in the community and the organist and the choir, sent to be Christ in the world for one another. I needed that. I don't need to be a tourist. I needed to be nourished and to be sent. And, I was.

It seems such a little thing to accompany a friend on her journey, yet in the midst of it all my journey continues. I am incredibly thankful for the invitation....and for the gifts of community and mission that were given in worship.

At odds and ends
Posted Nov 1, 2012 12:01 p.m.

A collection of contrasts and completed projects and conundrums.

1) My next set of scans and lab work are scheduled on Tuesday, November 13.

2) I am in preparation for leading the "Seven Spiritual Gifts of Waiting" class on Sunday mornings at St. John's Lutheran in Rock Island, and on Wednesday evenings at First Lutheran in Rock Island. It isn't a secret that I am leading these classes. I've been asked to by those pastors and I

appreciate the opportunity to participate in this bit of ministry. However, I am not interested in "sheep stealing" in any way....this is a conundrum to me, and if I let it, it can take some of the joy out of this leading. Unlike most pastors who leave one call, I have not gone to another call "far away" from the first. I am still here in town and am thankfully still close to my local friends and great medical care. I am still praying for the dear folks at Trinity and I know they are praying for me. For the sake of that ongoing wonderful ministry at Trinity, I will not invite former parishioners into my next ventures. However, I respect that the pastors and congregations that I teach or lead in next will not close their classes or worship to "members only" (this is about loving the neighbor, not shutting the neighbor out). This is a wonderful study and I am already encouraged by it and find great hope in it, as I wait and wait on the Lord.

3) We had over 75 trick or treaters last night and it was a fantastic night due to the last minute addition of PlayDoh to distribute! Woohoo! I just love hearing those kids walk away and say to their folks "Hey! I got PlayDoh!" Here's to more creative time spent together in families.

4) The left grey wool cabled fingerless mitten is about 60% done. Thanks be to God. I will attribute the last 20% of that project (a particularly tricky 20%) to the Hurricane Sandy storm. I was having a hard time figuring stuff out and dropped a stitch or two and the pattern was off by two stitches. Then, an east coast neighborhood lost 80 homes to fire. I started knitting again. This is just a mitten.

5) In our family, November has been pretty tough these last years. Rod died in 2004 and our nephew Joe Brines (a senior in college) died in 2010 on Thanksgiving weekend. Today on this All Saint's Day, I give thanks for these two saints, with much love and longing. It is November, and sometimes it is just more so.

It's complicated. It's simple.
Posted Nov 5, 2012 11:07 a.m.

Today is the eighth Anniversary of Rod's death from colon cancer at age 46. Years ago, when the first leaf turned colors for fall, I would enter a funk that I didn't emerge from until December. After a while the "season" decreased from October to November. Now it is pretty much just November.This year my grief is more complicated. A year ago I was still very overwhelmed by my diagnosis and was only a few weeks into my recovery from the tumor removal surgery when this anniversary came up. This year, much more clear headed, I am feel a bit like I am making "grief soup" (....to note, there is a wonderful children's/adults' book called "Tear Soup" which I recommend). I have added to this soup, tears, fears, some anger, some hope, frustration, determination, faith, courage, more tears, remembrance of joys, napkins (because the tissues are never on the dining room table), and time.

I have dealt with this cancer, knowingly, for over a year now. That helps me feel stronger than the cancer. Rod dealt courageously with his for six months and six days. We both have had attitudes that have compelled us to give our best selves to what ever we do. This includes striving for healing here and now, with the promise of ultimate healing in God's eternity.

Ready....and waiting
Posted Nov 10, 2012 4:58 p.m.

I had a bit of scanxiety last week. Most likely I will get a bit more of that, however, not today. It seems like you all are "pre-praying" me through my day with lab work (7:15 a.m.), MRI (7:30 a.m.), CT Scan (8:45 a.m.), orthopedic surgeon visit (11:00 a.m.) and oncologist visit (11:45 a.m.) next Tuesday, November 13. I can't begin to tell you what a gift that is. It truly keeps me more calm and trusting -- and more able to seem the Spirit at work in the midst of every day.

Woohoo!
Posted Nov 13, 2012 2:40 p.m.

Are you ready for this? Everything looks great in the hip. The tumors in the lungs may even be ever so slightly smaller. Woohoo!!! Thanks be to God.

Breathing...and sorting
Posted Nov 14, 2012 11:16 a.m.

Just yesterday afternoon, Mom and Dad and I were sitting in the doctor visit/exam room in Oncology. I had had lab work. I had two scans, I had a visit with Dr. Buckwalter where he said that my hip still looked good -- no cancer re-occurrence there. Then, we wandered on to the Cancer Center. I began knitting on the right mitten for Erica, having finished the left one while I was waiting to drink that odd purple contrast medium drink for the CT scan.

 One of my former research nurses came out to greet us in the waiting area, and to let us know that Dr. Mo had a really busy clinic day, and not to worry about the extra waiting.

An hour or so later we were called back. The med. tech. asked her usual questions and left. The door was open, as if even the door was hoping "bring good news...bring good news."

Dr. Mo walked by once, then once again and looked at me as he was moving by the door on the way to another patient and said, "Your scans look good!" I cheered out. I started to cry. I think Mom and Dad started to cry, too. I couldn't believe it. Part of me still can't. I said to them, "We are praying. I ask for stuff all the time....I am going to say thank you."

So....we prayed.

When Dr. Mo came in to see us, he told us that he tries to let people who are waiting know about their good news if he can, because he knows it is hard to wait. Certainly it was helpful to me because I got some good (happy) crying out of the way and was better able to hear what he had to say when he came back in the room. It was fun to see him cheerful, too.

I had other questions beyond just the tumor information, and my folks and Dr. Mo seemed to keep telling me something like --"You get it that the tumors are stable-- right?" I did get that. Or maybe not, as it seemed way too good to be true. I wanted to ask him about the shortness of breath and some pain in my chest, which he explained was a result of the fluid in the pleural effusion around my lungs. It doesn't seem to worry him. He could tell that I needed to actually see the scan, so he pulled up the current and the August scan on the computer screen in the room and compared three of the larger tumors which he described as slightly smaller. He described the rest as "stable." Basically he told me to just keep doing whatever I was doing because it was working.

In my mind I was thinking through what I was doing....eating, drinking water, eating cookies, lots of prayer, exercise/physical therapy, prayer, teaching, worship, prayer, enjoying my family and friends, lots of knitting, more praying....I love all these things...I can do this. It feels like he just gave me November 13 through February 13, wrapped them with a bow, and set them on my lap. Oh my, how beautiful. What a season of thanksgiving this is.

It felt good to be able to walk all those halls with my parents yesterday...pretty much keeping a normal pace. That is so very different from a year ago when I had just moved from a walker to a cane to get around home and was a long way from being able to walk those long halls in Iowa.

At home last night I was pretty sore....which was not unexpected after all the walking and two days of travel. Probably I was just as emotionally exhausted as I was physically exhausted. Because the support you all provide is so very important to me and my family, I wanted you to know more about how yesterday's good news came about.

Quiet...and acutely aware
Posted Nov 21, 2012 10:33 a.m.

Today....there is lament.

I was about to go to bed and I started stewing. Just two words did it: "compression atelectasis." Two words from my radiologist's final interpretation of my lung CT. The fluid in the pleural effusions, (fluid that has developed in between the two layers of tissue that surround the whole lung field) has pressed on my lower left lobe and caused this atelectasis (little alveoli that flatten out and don't fill with air when I inhale). I started ruminating on everything I could think of to get those little air sacs to get with the party. The stress was going to keep me from sleeping well. So, I decided to do what I promised myself I would do when all this mess started over a year ago -- I would ask Dr. Mo.So, at 10:40 p.m. last night I emailed him. That didn't seem quite enough so I asked a nurse friend to read the report and pray as well. I anticipated I would hear from Dr. Mo in the morning. Ten minutes later he emailed back. Basically he said, "no worries...it is ok....this can happen" and some simple things to try. My nurse friend said the same...and she prayed....and I slept. That darkness is so close some times -- as is the lament that goes with it. A few weeks ago, probably 2-3 weeks before my scans, the "scanxiety" had me in that same dark place. When I was "there," I was journalling and wrote the following prayer...

Lord, Please stick with me here. When I am in this pit, I know you are holding me. The only way to look up and out is through your embrace. I push aside the robe...I see your smile...a nod that it will be ok. I rest back down. The pit is ok if You are here. Help me get this lament out of me. If it is out, perhaps it can stay out and not come back. In Hope's name, I pray, Amen.

I'm not in the same place now, and I am thankful for that. However, I acutely aware of many folks who are there right now. Folks for whom the Thanksgiving-Advent-Christmas time is not only dark outside...it is dark inside, for a variety of reasons. I, with many others, wish we could take that darkness away. I hope that in that darkness, all can see the Light who is there, hearing our lament....banishing darkness...

Hope
Posted Nov 29, 2012 2:33 p.m.

It is a quiet noon here at home. The sound of the high efficiency washer and the furnace battle it out for the quietest loudness. I read my way through a chapter on Compassion for my class as I munch on a half of a ham sandwich and some raw veggies. I offset my health food with a Diet Pepsi. The author (Holly Whitcomb) says that while we are waiting, the compassion offered to us can give us hope. I look at a small note in the margin of my book. "Todd look @ cars w/ Rod" My head flooded with that memory. Rod was on chemo. Things weren't looking so good. Rod was thinking about how we were going to manage in the fall with a new driver in the house (Erica about to turn 16) and only two cars. He figured if he got a "new old car" that Erica could drive his newer, safer car. He was determined to look for used cars. The thing was, he couldn't drive any more. Todd, his friend, would take him out to look at cars. I found out later that he even drove at least one of them. At the time I was frustrated by this. I really could NOT see how we would be able to afford a new car as we were trying to get by on my salary and his $100.99 per week disability payment. (Really...what a joke.) I was worried about everything.I look back now.Looking at those cars gave Rod hope. It helped him feel normal. It helped him stay in the game of life. It helped him be a dad. It got him out of the house for something that felt good -- friendship and laughter -- time with the guys. Hope. A few years later, when I made that note in the margin, I had remembered that compassion and was thankful.

Now, however, I get it. I wish I had understood the power of that simple act of Todd's to give so very much. Today, I am wearing my LiveStrong HOPE shirt. It is Advent now. It is a season of hope and promise and now I get it.My "used car" hope is this class I am teaching. It reminds me that that although death is at work, life is ever more at work. Just because part of me is sick doesn't mean all of me is sick. Just because part of me is differently-abled, there is still so much of me that is very able. I give thanks for the compassion of my pastor friends and their congregations who have given me this gift of hope. It is the most beautiful Advent gift I have ever received.

Today, I so want to give that gift of hope to my nephew Joe's mom and dad....and to his brothers and their families. Two years ago today, Joe took his own life. The more I try to sort out what deep sadness Joe was in, the less I can figure it out. The only thing I can do is to look forward. To name the sadness. To walk along side them in their sadness, with compassion. Hopefully, while walking together, we can hear what the Psalmist says about the Spirit present with us always, and stay with us, even in our deep griefs. (Psalm 139)*Where can I go from your Spirit?where can I flee from your presence?If I climb up to heaven, you are there,If I make the grave my bed, you are there also.If I take the wings of the morningand dwell in the uttermost parts of the sea,Even there your hand will lead meand your right hand hold me fast.*

This "used car hope," this "teach a class hope," this "walk along side hope" is coming....the manger is waiting.

The days of the lost Mary
Posted Dec 1, 2012 10:18 a.m.

Advent preparations are pretty much complete here at home. All of our manger scenes are displayed -- with all of the baby Jesus figures in the drawer in the living room.There is only one problem. The Little People plastic Mary is AWOL. How is it that I can keep track of 50+ camels to add to that set, but have lost Mary? This troubles me. (Never trouble a theologian with a mixed up manger scene.)

Day 1 of the lost Mary: Searched all of office stuff from church, as this is where she was last used in display. Searched all of camel herd....they aren't talking.

Day 2 of the lost Mary: I go for a walk. My mind is filled with "Mary thoughts." I see a mother with two children coming toward me. I wonder if she is my "Mary." One of the two children is walking way ahead of the mom and little sister. The kids are preschool age. Mom is *not* happy about the racing ahead. She shouts out "GAVIN MICHAEL!" She is serious! I decide that she is not Mary, and probably GAVIN MICHAEL is John the Baptist. A block later I see another Mom. She is carrying armloads of children's clothing on hangers from a house to the hatch of a car. There is a little girl in the doorway of the house. There is some stress on her face as she goes back and forth with clothes....I think that mom is Mary. I don't tell her she is not in my scene in my living room. She is busy with her child. I turn the corner and see three Rock Island track team members running from East to West on 18th Avenue; yep, three wise men. (They probably don't need camels as they were very good runners.) I go home. I love my neighborhood manger scene.

Day 3 of the lost Mary: I go to walk again and listen to a preaching podcast. The podcast was about preparing to preach for the first Sunday in Advent. I didn't see any of my neighborhood nativity scene, although, I saw many many people in cars. I think they were traveling places so they could be taxed.

Later on Day 3: I go to the Christmas at Augustana concert and the smorgasbord that preceded it. Chaplain Richard Priggie, in his remarks solved my Mary dilemma. He quoted the German mystic Meister Eckhart, but I'll just summarize the Chaplain. He said we are all Mary -- you, me, that Mom, my neighbor. Christ is born in all of us. Not just the girls. Not just the boys. We all get to bear Jesus. If we don't, then we miss Jesus with us now. Right now.

Day 4 of the lost Mary: I am still bugged by losing one of the crucial pieces of my Fisher Price Manger Scenes. I am still going to look for her. I still have time because Jesus doesn't come out of the drawer for another 24 1/2 days. In the mean time, I'm going to remember that I get to be Mary.

The mittens
Posted Dec 4, 2012 12:33 p.m.

They are done. The grey wool fingerless cabled mittens are done. By five rows into the second mitten I was having fun. I couldn't believe it. It turns out that it isn't so hard to knit when I know how. Most of the most recent frustration came this morning when I tried to post a little slide show to Facebook of the mitten "process," from my practice knitting with double pointed needles on green yarn, to the finished mittens last evening. Facebook finally let me post a video of this project.

Technological frustrations aside, I am quite delighted to have had this project. Why? Because:
1) I was able to delight my daughter with these mittens.
2) Prior to this point, she knew I loved her because I painted the trim in her bedroom (there was a LOT of trim)....and of course put her though college, but she notes the trim thing as #1.3) I was reminded that even complex, insurmountable challenges can be overcome with practice, patience, prayer and more of all three.
4) When I see the mitten, I think of my mom and my Grandma Davis who do and did beautiful work in what ever they attempted. Many times they did so for me.
5) It helps me feel "productive."
6) It was worth doing....even if it had turned out poorly, it was worth doing just to share the love.

7) it reminds me that I'm still being knitted....some is, and some isn't; a pattern of my own choosing, but I trust the Knitter.

Better or worse
Posted Dec 5, 2012 2:27 p.m.

I've been pondering what makes life better or worse.
The next thing I'll mention is definitely a better for me and for my family in the long-term, even though it might seem quite odd to you -- even if just in the sense that very few people talk about it. I started a list of scripture, liturgy, and hymns/songs that I would like used at my Celebration of Life (funeral). I have thought of that for many many years as a pastor -- and while providing pastoral care to countless families at the time of a death. Rod and I talked about that during his illness. He shared and I shared. I wrote down his choices, but he wasn't in a position to record my choices. None-the-less, I never wrote down that stuff for myself.
There are a couple of reasons to do that now: I feel pretty good. I can think clearly. I have cancer (although this is not necessary for writing this stuff down). I can type. When stuff comes to mind it is easier to add to a list if a list is already started. It is important to me. This stuff (the Bible stories, the liturgy, the music and lyrics) will all be a part of my confession of faith -- my witness -- when I am not there to speak it.
Now, I'll admit that short-term I feel a bit worse. It makes me so sad to imagine the sorrow of my family. However, in the long-term, this is definitely a better. It feels better having it done. It is less stressful for me than repeatedly telling myself "I should do that." I will have it done, and I will keep a copy of this list where I keep my will.

This is not a unique or rare event I am planning for. We *all* get one. The big party that I'll be attending while people are following my notes is one that has already been planned, has already started, and will be going on long after I catch up to it.It is ok to write up the stuff that is important on a "better" day. Honestly, it is a "this will help you someday" sort of a gift to my family, and I do like gift-giving.

197

Angels...and a little bit of heaven

Posted Dec 14, 2012 2:53 p.m.

While a new Mary has been placed in the stable, it is angels I see today.

In my collection of treasured Christmas decorations are two crocheted angels made by my Grandma Lucille Davis. At the heart of the word, angel, is the notion of being a messenger -- particularly a messenger of good news.

I thought about angels last night as I attended the Lessons and Carols service at Augustana College's Ascension Chapel. The bell choir was only four songs into the performance and I already had tears coming down my cheeks. It was remarkable, actually, heavenly.

I've heard of people who have had experiences where they perceive they have died and then returned to life. If what I heard from those bells and voices last night is anything at all like the song of heaven, I can see why people would not want to return. The musicians and directors' gifts are truly heaven sent.

I had some other thoughts on angels, but right now they pale in comparison with my desire to offer Good News to the people who are effected by the elementary school shooting in Newtown Connecticut. The whole world wants to take away the deep pain of this day -- to return the children and teachers to their families and communities. Lord, have mercy.

The Good News that I know, is that God has chosen to make a home with us....in us...and in the community of the church. God be with them, and all of us.

In the middle...
Posted Dec 15, 2012 9:01 p.m.

On December 14, twenty children and six adult staff members were shot at Sandy Hook Elementary School in Newtown, Connecticut.
In the middle...
of the nation's grief...
of Advent...
of a rainy day...
Rod's sweet mother, Dorothy Elaine Koppenhoefer,
entered eternal life…
in the middle of the all the saints, especially her husband and son and grandson,
in the middle of God's love
in the middle of our thoughts
in the middle of our prayers of thanksgiving...
for this life well lived and loved in God's grace....

Something so small
Posted Dec 20, 2012 10:08 a.m.

It's not quite Christmas yet. The Gospel for Advent 4 (Luke 1:39-55 this coming Sunday) has expectant Mary coming to visit her expectant cousin Elizabeth. And the most remarkable small thing happens; baby John in Elizabeth's womb kicks when he hears Mary's voice. It's just a little thing, really, but Elizabeth knows God is at work, and says so. The later part of this reading is what has come to be called The Magnificat (my soul magnifies the Lord). Even when the Lord is seen at work in the smallest of ways, our souls swell with hope and promise.

Even in these last days of sadness after Elaine's death, small things remind us of an ever present God....

~ an afternoon with Sarah where we made 20 dozen springerle...her wearing her Grandma Koppenhoefer's apron for the first time.

~ Enough time at my parent's home to relax, bake more cookies, and decorate our version of Gingerbread houses.

~ Time spent telling stories of Grandma Koppenhoefer...and of Grandpa Roger Harding, who died one year ago yesterday.

~ The news of a little baby born, over 2000 years ago, announced to shepherds and their sheep, would be the Son of God...ever present....

- The Spirit of the same God who remains with the countless grieving in Newtown Connecticut and around the nation.

With love and thanks
Posted Dec 23, 2012 10:11 a.m.

The coffee is hot and sweet. The furnace blows air through these big 80-year-old vents...one beside me. The tree lights shine even brighter than the sun in my Sunday-morning-lit living room. The tissues beside me get a work-out, from tears of thanksgiving.

The 4th Sunday is Advent is favorite of mine. I am reminded of my Holy Land trip two and a half years ago. One of my favorite works of art is a sculpture of pregnant Mary and pregnant Elizabeth greeting one another that is displayed outside of the Church of the Visitation in Ein Karem, west of Jerusalem in Israel. In it is captured the joy of shared experience, the love of family, the hope of things to come, the promise of God, the miracle of ongoing creation, and of God turning everything upside-down....which is reflected in Mary's song....the Magnificat.

A year ago for me, the cancer was growing. The chemotherapy trial had started. The wounds from my hip surgery and port placement were still tender and new. I walked with a cane when I was out just to make sure I didn't land in a heap on the ground. And, many medications were needed just to making it through the day.

This year those wounds are well healed. The cane is gathering dust. The pain is managed with medication and physical therapy. The tumors are present but not growing...one even showed off by "backing off a few millimeters". I am daily lifted in prayer by more people than I can count. Even in the line at the visitation for my mother-in-law countless people shared that they continue to pray for me.

This year I have taken on making more of the gifts than I ever have in my life. Some of that may be a function of the time that I have, but I think that more of it is the thanks and gratitude I have for my family and friends. I want them to know that their love and care makes all the difference in the world to me. Their love is evidence that God is here. Making those gifts helps me "be here now."The desire to be here for many many seasons is quite strong. Unfortunately, when I spend time imagining those Christmas times ahead, I also get worried. That sort of emotion is inevitable....however, it isn't a fun place to stay.So, for now I return to the visitation of Mary to Elizabeth....present for and with one another. Thankful for the gifts of love between them and from God. Thankful for God who is turning everything upside down.May the hungry be fed....may the rulers be just....may the needs of the lowly be lifted up....may the poor be given good things....and may we all be healed on the journey.

Holding, being held...
Posted Dec 24, 2012 2:18 p.m.

Twenty years ago on this night, a 31-year-old me, and a 6-week-old Sarah, in a "Mary costume" and in swaddling clothes sat in a manger scene in our church, amongst a large cast of people playing other roles. The live goat in the scene munched on the hem of my dress. My parents "beamed" brighter than the stars in the sky (and prayed that the candles that people held in the pews wouldn't ignite the hay in the scene). Rod played guitar and Erica sang with the children. That night, Jesus became real to me in a new way....in a "this sweet child came for the world...and was loved by Mary and Joseph in ways that they couldn't even begin to express in words....and loves us back with an even more perfect love". Holding her...loving God...loving her. I could have sat there all night.

When I pray, I try to remember that holding and being held. When I pray, I take both of my hands, palms up, and lay one on top of the other. With the top hand, I experience being held. With the bottom hand, I practice holding.

That is what we all get to do this night: hold the Christ Child and be held by him. That is what we can do each day. With each sharing of the peace,

with each gift given,with our offerings to those in need, with each embrace in these days....we hold that Christ Child closely. With each sorrow lifted up, with each grief shared, with each tear shed, with each prayer prayed, and with each sigh offered when words are done, we are held securely in Christ's loving arms. These are gifts for each day... Thank you for holding me and those I love in Christ's healing embrace in this past year.

Learn a new thing...
Posted Dec 26, 2012 11:22 p.m.

The house is pretty quiet this day-after-Christmas. That is ok. Erica has been at work since 3:00 a.m. Sarah is in Morton to baby-sit some cousins. I am here...where it is quiet...remembering the wonderful sounds of the last two days.Like most days, I wanted to have it begin with some sort of scripture or study. I remembered that I had not heard all of Bishop Wollersheim's preaching on Youtube -- a video of his preaching for Trinity Lutheran's 100th anniversary celebration in December (the last of many steps of the celebration year). I wanted to hear the third point of his sermon. It was worth going back for. He described his yearly ice fishing exhibition to the Canadian-US boarder with a good friend....and the set up of an elaborate ice fishing house on the lake. Once it was all set up, he said, it wasn't time to rest, it was time to fish. Then he looked around that beautiful sanctuary and told the worshipers and us all in whatever sanctuaries we have set up, that it isn't time to rest, it is time to fish.... Jesus called us to fish for people. Yep. I may be down, but I'm not out. I'm still fishing.

This year I learned new things in order to make most of my gifts. It will be a week before all of them are distributed, so I'm not describing them all here, but most had to do with baking, drawing, wrapping, or crocheting. The joy I have already received in making and giving these gifts almost defies description. The process helped me learn more about my family, my

202

friends, and myself as well.I think that a part of the "fishing' that we are called to do is most simply to be our best selves for the sake of others, in Jesus' name.

All the while I am doing this....I am praying that there are scientists and doctors and researchers and pharmacists and teachers and counselors and legislators and companies and churches and all communities--- all being their "best selves" and learning new things, so that cancers can be cured. So that people can be fed. So that people with mental illness can know hope. So that nations can be at peace. So that the grieving can be comforted. So that people can have meaningful work. For the sake of others. There is such joy in it. I am so glad I have learned new things. The Bishop is right. It is not time to rest, it is time to fish.

Singing for healing...
Posted Dec 31, 2012 12:34 a.m.

I am pretty conscious of my breathing...when something is going wrong, that is. I know what makes me short of breath. I am planning ahead for this very cold air and know that I will need to head out with a scarf to breath through. I know that being outside when it is cold makes what ever I am doing a bit harder to breathe in. I also know that many folks find these things to be true.

However, this morning, in a warm, sun-filled sanctuary, sitting with my friend, Penny, and surrounded by familiar faces, I had a wonderful "lung" experience. Often, on the Sunday after Christmas, the worship consists of a series of lessons (Bible readings which chronicle the Christ story up to his presentation in the temple at a few days of age) and carols (traditional Christmas hymns paired in meaning/relevance with the lessons). My first few worship services after my recovery from surgery and chemotherapy, I loved the singing, but didn't have much vocal reserve. Today I felt the opposite. I could and did sing every song.

Luther said those who sing, pray twice. That is what I did today. After the second song I had the strongest sensation that the worship today was a healing worship. Sometimes there is a laying on of hands with prayer and anointing. This wasn't that. It was simply the gift of song....the exercise of it....the beauty and poetry of the story....the voices raised together with the glory of the organ accompaniment.

I know that in my mind some time ago, I perceived Lessons and Carols as a bit of a cop-out. Where's the preaching? After I was a pastor I saw how helpful it could be to have a break on one Sunday in one of the busiest times of the year. Most pastors I know preach several Christmas services and usually have a few funerals around that time as well....that is just the way it is.

But today. Angels from the realms of glory, sang to a rose 'er blooming, while "Away in a Manger" Mary asked "What Child is This?" Joy... "Joy to the World"....and a gift to me in body, mind and spirit.

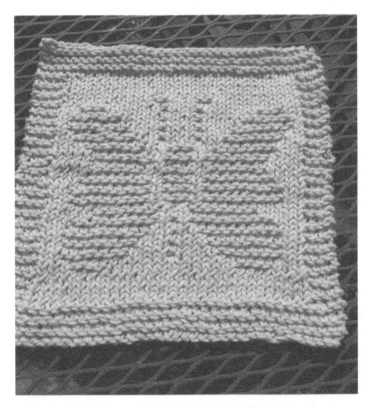

The butterfly washcloth. My first knitting project

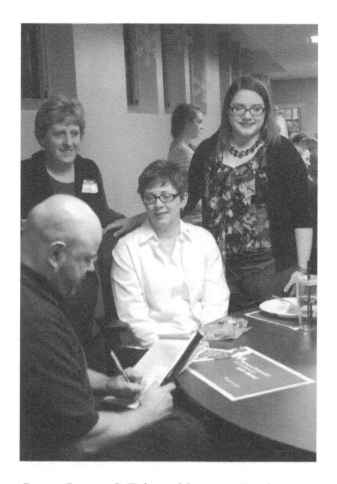

Penny Logan & Erica with me as I'm inter-
viewed by Stephen Elliott of the Moline
Dispatch/Rock Island Argus at the FUN-
draiser held for me at Trinity Lutheran
Church in Moline, Illinois. Over 500 people
attended to support me as I began a Chemo
Clinic trial.

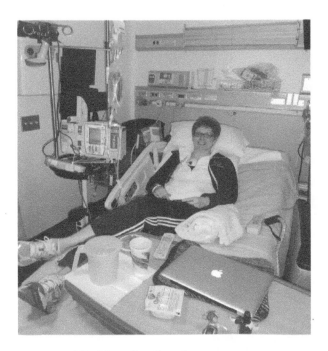

Waiting for the chemo

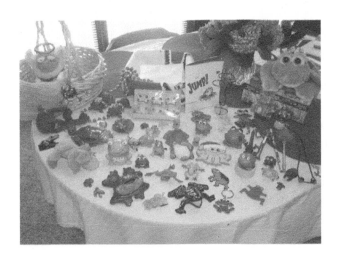

Frogs from around the world

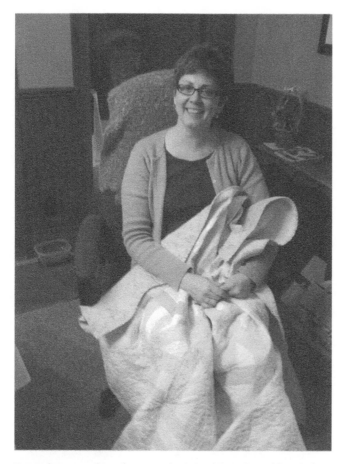

I am honored and overwhelmed by the gift of the
Sonshine Hope Quilt designed & made by Brooke
Witsberger. Brooke's gift was the first of many
beautiful & prayer-filled, hand-made gifts that
have kept me warm & loved through difficult days.

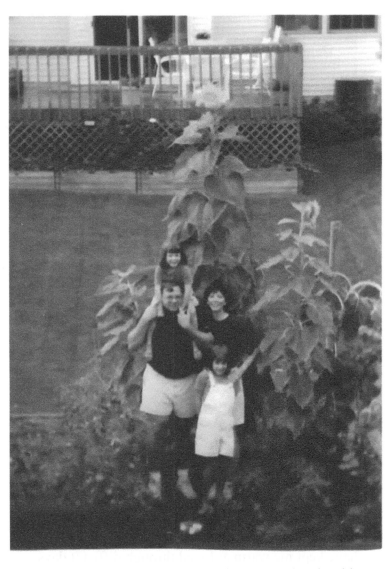

Summer Mid-1990's – Sarah sitting on Rod's shoulders
Erica in front of Laura

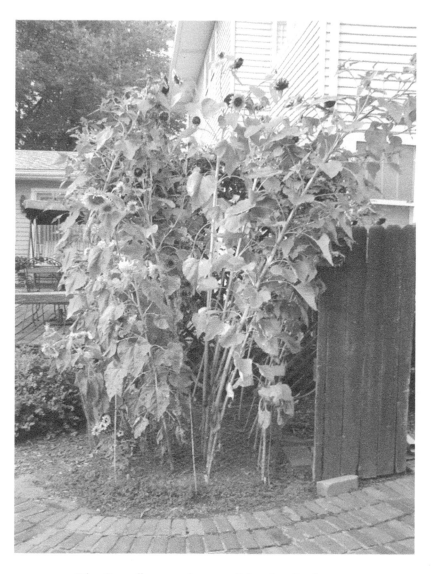

The "sunflower play-pen" by the deck

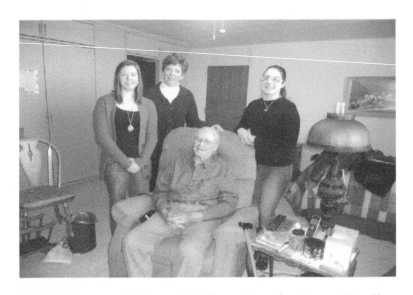

Sarah, Laura, and Erica with Great Grandpa Roger Harding

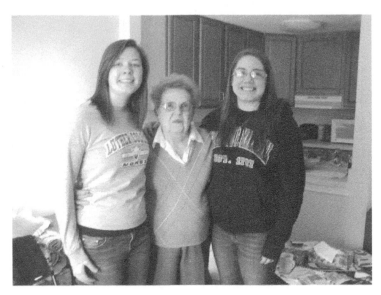

Sarah and Erica with Grandma Dorothy Koppenhoefer

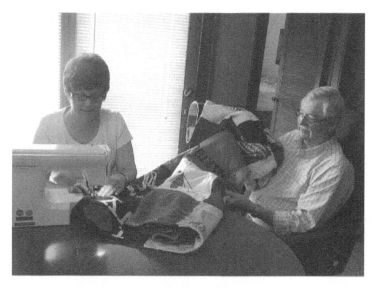

David Harding, Laura's father, helping Laura make a
t-shirt quilt for Sarah

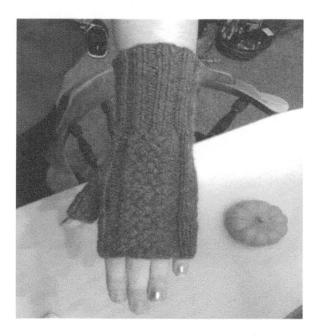

Erica models the left-hand-grey-wool-
cabled-fingerless-glove.

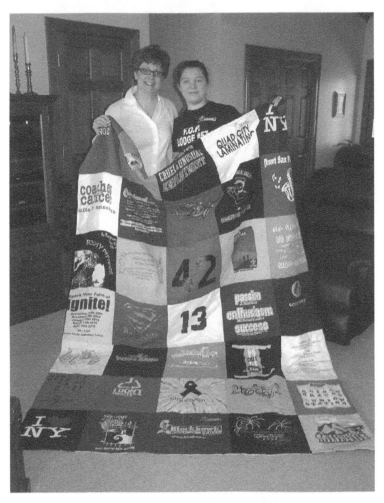

Laura & Sarah with Sarah's new t-shirt quilt

2013 UPDATES

Measuring...

Posted Jan 1, 2013 10:39 a.m.

It is New Year's Day, 2013. The sun is shining. Twenty birds, or so, are making a big deal of the 1/2 cup of bird food that I snuck into the feeders late yesterday. One-half cup is a big deal, but who's measuring. Me, of course.Thirteen months ago, growths of one to two millimeters on "many" tumors in my lungs started up solid full time work for myself and many others. So small, but bigger. One and a half months ago, one tumor was two millimeters smaller in one direction and three millimeters in another. The other tumors just voted "present." And, we all danced a jig.

This year, I slept through the Central Time Zone ball drop; however, I couldn't be happier. The new year stretches out the time from my own diagnosis to a very present "now." While the months "say" I am a 15-month survivor since diagnosis, the years vote a big, fat, life-filled "two." So, what might that add, if one were measuring? It adds the stuff one cannot measure....joy, hope, grace, thanksgiving, opportunity. I look back outside. A cardinal has joined the "1/2 cup feast." "There's plenty here," he says. But who's measuring?

Peace
Posted Jan 16, 2013 12:01 p.m.

The house sits quiet then,
as if its breath long held
releases its long warm sigh
through 80-year-old vents
pushing warm air on me
faster than these old cold closed windows still breeze in the January chill.

This peace longs for warm days and open windows.
I sit and wonder
about the peace found here
without a tree and lights
without gifts piled high
without wrapping and cards
without cookies spread out cooling in three rooms.
This after-it-all sort of peace is over-rated.

I check the calendar
and weigh the pull of today's chores
upcoming projects with friends
a concert a month away
and scans for tumors two-thirds of their way toward reassessment.
There is some peace to be found when I stay in "today."

The plants in the house
signal time for watering in this dry, warmed air,
but only one speaks.
An old Peace Lily has sent up the season's sentinel
in one erect bloom
facing not the window
facing not the table where we laugh and eat and bills are paid
facing the wall
facing only the wall which holds a Cross.
Silently speaking as loudly as it can

Peace comes not in a season
Peace comes not in quiet after busy times.
Peace comes not in one day or another.
This Peace, watered and blooming
knows peace only through the cross...
and One who claimed victory o'er
seasons
busy-ness
calendars
dis-ease
and death.
There is...
Here is...
Peace

Hope and the Wrestling Match
Posted Jan 24, 2013 11:02 a.m.

Do you ever find that a word, usually a simple one, when seen or written over and over suddenly becomes odd? The letters and their sounds and the word itself seem oddly disconnected. You might wonder if it is just a jumble of letters or if it really means something.

Or have you ever had the experience of having some sort of concept or idea that you believed in or about that suddenly seemed hallow or confusing? Did you ever question it? Did you question yourself and how you got there, to that odd place?

I'm asking these questions for a few reasons:
1) I don't think I'm alone in these wonderings.
2) Misery loves company.
3) And, I have come out on the other side of this wrestling, still wondering how I got into it in the first place.

Hope….Such a simple word. Yet it knocked me off of my theological feet for a few weeks.

I wanted "Hope" to be the theme of my Christmas cards and looked for five weeks for cards with that word on them. No luck. Then, I decided I would make some. However, by then I wasn't sure what hope was.

Was it...

~ I hope I get home before it starts to ice over outside?

~ I hope we get to see so and so for Christmas?

~ I hope that Sarah's books arrive from Amazon before she heads back to school. (They did not.)

~ I hope Sarah stays well at college. (She has had the stomach flu for several days now.)

~ I hope that those tumors stay tiny or get smaller or there is a cure or this is just a big, bad dream because another scan is less than a month away now....

Those questions feel more like dreams and wishes and that didn't feel like enough. I wanted to take hope by the shoulders and shake her and say, "Talk to me like you used to! What was it you used to say?"

I watched a video of a man who has stage-four cancer speaking at a friend's church. I know that someplace in his talk he mentioned hope. It was just a few words in the midst of a long speech. I had the thought that I would go back and listen.... Then I realized that even if it was "remarkable," that it was "his" way of understanding hope. I needed to figure this out for myself. However, it did help me move off dead center.

Not being able to define hope is a pretty lonely and scary place when cancer is in that place too. I didn't really want to talk about it either. I didn't want people worrying that I had "lost hope" and "worrying." When, actually I couldn't figure out hope, let alone find it. I wondered if I was just "thinking too hard," or if I was just now beginning to examine the core of what really mattered.

The self-applied pressure of sending some sort of a card for the Holidays kept pushing me along. Christmas had passed. New Years Eve/Day. Epiphany. Ground Hog Day and the "Season of the Annual Meeting" (for the pastor/lay leader types in this group) are almost here. Still, no way to talk about hope.

A friend shared some ideas from her thinking on Hope. "Hope is definitely not the same thing as optimism. It is not the conviction that something will turn out well, but the certainty that something makes sense, regardless of how well it turns out. Hope is a feeling that life and work have meaning." I figured that that helped. It wasn't everything about hope but it got me off a lonely center.

It got me to starting on that ol' card. I went to just making a list of what happened this year and then went to find those things in pictures....Rod's Mom's 90th birthday, making a quilt with Sarah, Erica's time as Maid of Honor, carving pumpkins....big things, little things, yearly things, once in a life time things. Seeing those pictures helped me. Those were not just things I hoped would happen -- they really did! It helped me remember those things that weren't in pictures as well....the joyful and the sorrowful, but all a part of truly living this past year. I remembered that *Faith, hope, and love abide*....(1 Corinthians 13). Really, they did. Some place in me, hope stirred. I made the card. It included Lamentations 3:21-23 as well. On the day the card went into the mail, another friend visited. She wondered this...and I paraphrase: "That it isn't only that we have hope in God, but God has hope in us. We are God's hope in the world." It had me remembering that hope isn't something that I only "have," it is something I do and live, as well.

I realized that for me, I had to know hope as something bigger that my circumstances and more effective than how my meds were working on a particular day and more reliable than whether or not the Cubs were winning (although I will admit that the Cub stuff is a pretty effective training ground for handling life's major/minor disappointments).
I don't think I'm done "figuring out" hope. However, I do know this: Hope is something God did (and continues to do). God took on flesh and dwelt among us, sending that sweet wriggling baby who was all wrapped up and laid in a manger -- Jesus, God's hope and our hope for the world. Similarly, hope is something I "do" as well, more than "have."

Not only on Sundays...
Posted Jan 27, 2013 12:40 p.m.

For many months I have not written on Sundays. It is the Sabbath. But then today, Sunday, I am at home rather than at worship. There is a sheen of ice on everything this morning. And, even the "thought" of falling on the ice, let alone difficulty driving to and from worship, have kept me at home, sipping tea, praying, reading, and looking out the windows to the back yard What am I reading? *Making Sense of the Cross* by David J. Lose. I will start leading a class on this book starting next Sunday, and a week from this Wednesday. Besides looking forward to doing this little bit of teaching, I was looking forward to the study. Then the book and resources came and I wasn't so sure. Was this going to be too "head" oriented with too little "heart"? Was it going to be all about history with little mystery? I wasn't sure. I started reading and getting engaged with the "dialog." (The entire book is a dialog.)

I don't mind looking out at my new deck and lawn. It is fine to look at. However, some day I will want to be outside. And if I am outside I will want to see what is growing. And if I see things growing, I will want to tend them. And if I really want to tend them, I will have to have some help. And if help comes (and I know it will), there will be a wonderful beautiful growing space that I will want to share with others. And when those people come and look at it, we will visit, and enjoy it, and share how somethings are hard to grow and some things are easy to grow and how we love the seasons and the tree that used to be there and what is new here.

And I miss worship. I can drive by the church during the week. I can see the Bibles on the big bookshelf in my living room. But I really miss them if I don't go into them. I miss the people and the stories and the growing and struggling, and the help when I need it, the seasons and the sharing.

This book is wonderful. It helps me, and I will help others move from "just watching through a window" to going inside our faith, asking questions, showing up to help one another, wondering about the seasons of our lives and what used to be there and what is there now, and how through the looking/wondering/questioning we get stronger muscles and sharper minds. These will serve us well in all sorts of weather. In all sorts of seasons.

Dust to dust
Posted Feb 13, 2013 10:23 a.m.

Today is Ash Wednesday. Lent begins. I've been praying about what my Lenten discipline(s) would be for some time now. I've decided to give up one thing and to do something each day that could be considered "being good to myself." The thing to give up was simple to figure out -- I am giving up using my iPhone once I go to bed. I am a little more connected to that electronic device than I need to be. I will still use it's clock/alarm/phone functions....and will still be accessible for emergencies by phone or text, but I will not "wile away the hours" by virtual wandering through Facebook and Pinterest at bedtime. There should be much more time for prayer, reading and sleep. This is good.

Last year I was recovering from a particularly horrible chemotherapy experience/hospitalization and preparing for chemotherapy #3 when Ash Wednesday rolled around. I missed the worship with the community. It is humbling and necessary to stop every so often and remember that I am dust, and to dust I shall return. It will be no surprise. That is the way of life and death. That I/we spend these days or years with life breathed into us is a gift.

Dancing
Posted Feb 14, 2013 11:53 a.m.

Day #2 in Lent. This morning, I exercised on my own. I decided to go dancing....Dancing with the Word, that is, using my friend and colleague, Rev. Janet Hunt's blog site "Dancing with the Word." I read her post about Jesus in the wilderness, his temptation. And, I am reminded of how I sort that out....the devil "tempts" with the expectation of one's failure. Jesus (like all good teachers) "tests" with the expectation of success. He can do that, because he has already taken the test, passed it, and given us the

219

answers. I love that kind of test. Jesus doesn't just expect us to walk with him.....he knows we can. I know I can. Better yet, let's dance.

"I'll take one and three, please."
Posted Feb 15, 2013 5:03pm

The best medicine today, started at 4:30 a.m. At 5:30, we (Steve, Sue and I) were out the door from their home and headed to Glen Ellyn, Illinois. By 8:00 a.m. we were greeting two of my sweet great-nephews -- ages one and three. I am confident that this is the very best way to spend this day: trains, books, Peter Pan, snacks, Lambie, monkeys, and fixin' things. Many hugs and kisses. All good. (Come Sunday evening I get to enjoy another set of great-nephews -- ages six and eight.)

Curving in...curving out
Posted Feb 17, 2013 12:29 a.m.

One problem with severe illness, or chronic illness, or life-threatening illness, or depression, or just being "ordinary-common-cold kind of sick," is that I (we, you, etc) tend toward a sort of mental, physical, and/or spiritual posture that is "curved in" on oneself. "Incurvatus en se" (in the Latin) This can be life-preserving, in some ways. It is also so very isolating. It can keep a person from being exposed to germs, I guess, but it also keeps one from living life.
Augustine, and later, Martin Luther, describe sin as being turned in on oneself. The resurrected life means standing again, forgiven, able to see the needs of the other, and breathing, being curved outward toward God, rather than inward toward self.
That brings me to these days. These busy days before my scans. In these sorts of days at other times, I have found myself "incurvatus en se"" to the point of practically being a human sized rollie-pollie. This sub-consciously/semi-consciously planned several days of travel and time with family is one of my statements against life shaped like a bubble. I remember a year ago, and how small my world felt, when I was awake enough to feel a world beyond my nausea. One of the gifts of living AND

220

being alive for it is to engage the world -- to live for someone's sake besides one's own. ....to teach a class, to make a Lutheran World Relief quilt, to vote, to pay my taxes, to pray for my neighbor, to recheck the applicability of gravity (reaffirming that the world does not revolve around me).

24 hours
Posted Feb 18, 2013 9:25 p.m.

In the last 24 hours, I have found joy in....
good meals with family
creating an obstacle course for my great nephew's remote control cars
touring Johnson Floral in Morton (my nephew/niece's wonderful business)
making it home in time to exercise
receiving many voice mail messages, letters, and emails of encouragement
receiving wonderful visits from two friends who both prayed with me
and having had a great meal out to eat with my family.
In the next 24 hours, I will receive care through your prayers and mat carrying
the nurses, techs, and MRI/CT staffs
my dear parents, my dear daughters (at home and at college)
and, Dr. Mo and Dr. Buckwalter.

Whew! And thank God and thank you
Posted Feb 19, 2013 5:55 p.m.

The view is good heading back east to Rock Island.... The news is good too. The tumors are ALL stable. There are no new tumors. There is a very slight increase in size of the left pleural effusion and the one on the right is stable. We are waiting for a final reading on the MRI of the hip to make sure it is clear. There was no compression atelectasis at all-- I think the exercises are helping that. Woohoo! This means no chemo for at least three months!

Blankets, and sleeping with the enemy
Posted Feb 21, 2013 10:06 a.m.

What I want to tell you about is how truly lovely it is to use the prayer shawls, quilts, and blankets that such dear people and congregations have given me on this journey. What you do, with hands, needles, hooks, and yarn or thread and material -- makes a loving, God-filled difference.

However, I am a few days "out" from my scans and have a thought that keeps "hanging around me" that I would just as soon not continue thinking about.

These little tumors in my lungs are quiet. They are sitting there, stable, not growing. I am very thankful for that. However, I do not want them there. When I was talking with Dr. Mo this week, I asked him a few questions that started something like this, "A year ago, all I wanted was to get these tumors out of my body. I had surgery for the big one, but I really wanted the ones in my lungs to go. (The big one caused most of the pain, but the little ones cause most of the fear.) I understand now that I am better off just leaving them alone, but every so often I still wonder about just getting them out. How about ablation or wedge resection? (radiation or surgery)?" Then he responded with why that is a bad idea, and could make the cancer worse. Which, I knew, but needed to hear again.

You see, keeping those cells inside me feels like I am sleeping with the enemy. I don't carry anger at them so much for how they have messed up my life, but in the last few days I have been incredibly angry and hateful toward them for the impact on my daughters' lives and my parents, my brother, my extended family, Rod's family, my friends, and parishioners. I want them to go away. I want the cause of that pain to be over.

Last night in Lenten worship, though, I realized something. I was fooling myself if I thought that the cancer tumors were the only enemy that I have living in me. Here also resides doubt, and fear, and powerlessness, and the notion that "I can do this on my own." Every one of these can rob me of life as I hope to live it. God, as I know God, is bigger, more loving, more patient, more persistent, more encouraging, more life-giving and affirming, more hopeful, more present (living in all of me, not just my lungs), than any of my physical or mental enemies.

I take a deep breath. There is more love than despair. There is more peace than there are pieces of tumor. There is more hope than hatred. I think I will rest under a blanket or two for a while, now that I remember who is who.

"But" or "And"
Posted Feb 22, 2013 7:06 p.m.

I came home from Iowa City with good news on Tuesday,

BUT, I didn't have all of the news.
I had a long email conversation throughout the morning with Dr. Mo, and, learned that I have several tiny tumors growing in my hip, around the site of the former tumor. I talked to him about "taking these out,"

BUT, I have learned that surgery is not a good idea...too big a surgery, too hard to find the tiny tumors, too big a chance they would just grow back. Dr. Mo notes that this is time to enjoy! No growth in the lungs, feeling pretty good, and, no chemo. I had some moments this morning...not my favorite kinds of moments.

BUT, I had a lot of "AND" moments.

My family loves me,
AND prays for me.
I got to see a dear friend out of the blue in the grocery store,
AND got a hug.
I was in a protracted conversation with God,
AND got a wonderful devotion emailed to me from a dear cousin.

AND, I spent this day living with cancer,

AND this afternoon, after groceries, I studied in preparation for teaching my next class on Sunday.

AND this evening, Penny and I will get to sewing on our second Lutheran World Relief Quilt.

AND God's love, and grace, and hope, and comfort take up a lot more room in me than those tiny tumors in my hip and my lungs.
AND each day, your prayers and the Spirit's presence add to my strength and focus.

Things that help
Posted Feb 25, 2013 12:10 p.m.

So, in terms of things that help:
1) that Dr. Mo has given me his personal email and communicates directly with me. I can deal with "stuff" so much better knowing that if I am troubled, I can ask him directly, and he will tell me the straight scoop.
2) that God, has given me God's personal, direct, communication line (prayer) and helps me deal with the "stuff" Dr. Mo tells me.
3) that of late, I have been falling asleep with a Palm (sized) cross in my right hand....this gives me a particular focus when I am drifting off to slumber-land. It also reminds me that even as I am holding on, that I am being held on to.
4) that working to get on with my previously scheduled life; going out to dinner, playing the piano, having dinner made for me, folding laundry, worship, taking in a movie, watching the Oscars, helping a friend pick out drapery fabric, exercising using a modified version of Just Dance 4 on the Wii, prayer, and preparing for teaching/preaching.
If these things should fail, or should I need a longer list of life things to get on with, I can/will include making an alphabetized list of the spices in our cabinet, knitting, doing dishes, feeding the birds, telling my family and friends that I love them, eating fewer cookies and drinking more water.
5) Remembering Rodney today, on his 55th birthday. That brings many smiles. I know he would be proud of all of his girls.

"Today you will be with me in paradise."

Posted Mar 2, 2013 10:06 a.m.

I am now teaching the *Making Sense of the Cross* by David Lose class. We have been reading the passion accounts in each of the four Gospels. We have been learning more about what points the writers were trying to make to each of their respective audiences about who God is and what God is doing through Jesus. These days I find that I reach toward the very compassionate Jesus found in Luke's Gospel -- the One who on the cross looked to the repentant thief on the cross near his and said, *"Today you will be with me in paradise."* (Luke 23:43) While I am no rush to run to that particular Paradise, I am ever so thankful for the Spirit's presence in this one. This paradise that includes:

1) a 40 minute Skype with dear friends and their little grandson, followed by a two hour Skype with Sarah, who is learning American Sign Language on the side and is helping me learn a bit as well. Last night I tried hope, courage, and brave, as well as weird and help, and an old favorite, Amen.

2) a tremendous meal at the Moline Exotic Thai with Erica.

3) time spent admiring the birds on my deck as they feast on old bread, and as "Bob the Black Squirrel" feasts on old grapes and apple cores.

4) preparing to sew with Penny.

5) hearing from far away friends on the phone.

6) planning for spring break time with family.

7) the outpouring of continued prayers from so so many people.

The sun is shining on our six or so inches of snow. The house is warm. The coffee steamy. The day stretches out ahead of me. God is good, and so very near.

A little lost...
Posted Mar 6, 2013 11:58 a.m.

I still know my address. I know everything that is in my spice cabinet (Erica alphabetized it and I typed it up). I know more about my family history (because of a paper that Sarah is writing for a class in college). The roads are clear and getting better after yesterday's snow, so I'm sure I could leave home and find my way back. Yet, I've been a little lost.

Since sometime last week, I've spent my "spiritual time and energy" in these ways:

Praying a lot.

Prepping for the class I am teaching.

Playing favorite hymns on the piano.

Worshipping.

Wrestling with whether the cancer that is in me is a life-threatening (or life-changing or life-ending) disease, *or* a chronic illness, *or* a disease that manifests chronically.

This has taken a lot of time. And, it some ways it seems a moot point. But, in other ways not. To accept the chronic aspect of this cancer somehow feels like I've given up trying to get rid of it. To accept the chronic aspect of it takes me back to the feeling like I am sleeping with the enemy. I think the contemporary term might be frenemy. It also could help me just get on with life, and not worry so much sort of like, "Hey, it's a pain, but it's just a chronic illness." Although, folks with diabetes, arthritis, and the like probably don't feel much like they have "just another disease."

It is a good thing this isn't a contest.However, when I use any of those other adjectives on the front of "disease" (except chronic) it seems like there is a sort of logical end point -- either "all better" or "dead." It implies that one knows what that end point should be and when it would come. That just isn't the case.

So. I figured that pairing my "disease versus chronic illness" debate with my current study of the theology of atonement (what God did/accomplished for humanity on the cross, resulting in healing the relationship between God and humanity) was right on.

226

Today, I studied the parable of the prodigal son (or "the really gracious dad" or "the really ticked off older brother").

And, I remembered that I can be lost, and still be right at home. I had wondered why I didn't have anything to write for a week, and I think it was because I was only listening to the stuff that was going on in my own head, and not listening for God.

So, this is what I think about the disease versus chronic illness thing. It doesn't matter. Not right now. I think that this particular wrestling is a distraction. It plunges me into worry. It keeps me from fully living, and fully living is very very important to me. I was a little lost there.

Turn around...
Posted Mar 8, 2013 9:37 a.m.

If I am looking for a straight line, I can use my quilt making ruler, or the tracks in the snow of "Bob the Squirrel" from the redbud tree to the ornamental pear tree.

If I am looking for a line that goes out a ways and then turns back, I can look at myself, in Lent. That's what Lent is about -- another chance to repent, to turn around, to turn back towards God. Lent is working on me.

The technology ban in bed at "bed time" and "wake up time" has me going to sleep earlier and waking on my own, more rested in the morning. Reading scripture "for my own good" each morning, has me seeing myself and the world more clearly through Spirit shaped eyes.

Regardless of what hurts on any given day, turning around has made everything feel better.
Today, Erica and I travel to Illinois State, and then turn around and bring Sarah home for a week. Spring Break. Those words sound beautiful.

227

So like the soil...
Posted Mar 9, 2013 10:58 a.m.

So like the soil
my soul longs for Easter.
For water it waits
dying and rising
renewed and stretching
open and gasping
sputtering
breathing.

Its harvest made
this ground sat hard and full of roots
dry and done.

To great sleeping fields
rains came
soaking deep within.
Then froze
and broke apart old paths.
Leaving room for something new.

Today the frozen earth
begins its thaw
and adds the weight of winter rain.
Waiting. Waiting.

All those weeks were sleeping, dying.
Now, the winter-Lenten land prepares for Easter.
For after dying comes the rising.
For after soaking comes the seed.
After planting comes the growing.
After growing comes the blooming
feeding
life and living.

With my eyes
I see it coming.
With my soul
I see the need.
With my heart
I wait rejoicing
hope for Easter,
hope for living
hope for life
for spring
and Thee.

Hope needs a kick-start

Posted Mar 21, 2013 10:01 a.m.

So, when a dear friend asks how I am doing and I start crying, maybe it is time to ask for some help. It seems that the now one-month-old news of the tiny tumors in my hip, combined with the cancer re-occurrence in a church friend has blurred my "focus." I'm not trying to deny what is going on, but I could use some prayers to focus on the truly awesome life that I have.

This morning I went to Romans (5:1-5)

Therefore, since we are justified by faith, we have peace with God through our Lord Jesus Christ,
2 through whom we have obtained access to this grace in which we stand; and we boast in our hope of sharing the glory of God.
3 And not only that, but we also boast in our sufferings, knowing that suffering produces endurance,
4 and endurance produces character, and character produces hope,
5 and hope does not disappoint us, because God's love has been poured into our hearts through the Holy Spirit that has been given to us.

"Lean on me"

Posted Mar 25, 2013 10:30 a.m.

When the girls were toddlers through young elementary school age our bedtime routine (once they were actually in bed) included the following:
Reading a book

Singing a song

Praying prayers

Doing all of that took a while, but it was the favorite ritual nonetheless.

Babysitters or grandparents weren't always so sure about the "sing a song" part, but they always did their best. Rod's #1 go-to song was Bill Wither's classic, "Lean on Me."

Last week I had reached a tipping point of what was possible for me to carry. I didn't have any new news or symptoms but I had picked up plenty of worries and problems to solve -- so many so that the pile of things in my arms obscured my vision and my balance! Daily -- or frankly more often -- God and I have long conversations about this or that, and I had been having those conversations about those burdens.
However, I wouldn't set them down. I just kept talking about what I had in my arms. However, on that one morning, as I was getting ready to spend the day with a girl friend, I decided to do more than tell God about it, I decided to tell you, and ask for help. For me, that admission of worry, and asking for help was like an actual release of those burdens. Within the hour I felt physically and mentally better. My focus improved. My joy improved. I have had four or five of the most delightful days, and I thank you for your support. I know that prayer helps, but if I am unwilling to change my behaviors (e.g., worrying, taking on stuff I don't need to take on), there won't be much change. If you all were here right now, I would sing "Lean on Me" to you.

Please know that I hold you all in prayer as you:
struggle with recovery from surgery
rejoice with or await births in your families
journey though depression
do your physical therapy
try to find a diagnosis
wonder when to retire
learn about retirement
strive to offer your best ministry in your current or new call
study for examinations
shovel snow (really!)
look for a job (or a new job)
be a loving care-giver
weep
dance
grieve
pray
stretch
hope
journey through Holy Week
look for a cure.

Vision, and what is seen
Posted Mar 29, 2013 6:01 p.m.

A story in three parts.

On Monday I cleaned. This is always good to do, but I ramped it up a notch. Over the course of an hour or two, I vacuumed the eleven panels of slatted (closet and armoire) doors in my bedroom. I hadn't thought they were that bad, but honestly, they look remarkable now. Who knew that dust had such a lousy color? I can see what they look like now, and they look fine, just fine.
On Monday morning, while home alone and enjoying an early morning cup of coffee and *The Argus*, something went screwy with my vision. Was it a floater? Was something on my glasses? Did I have "sleep" in my

eyes? I couldn't tell which eye was the culprit. Then, as quickly as something started, it got better. That evening at supper time, something was odd again. This time Erica was there. She looked in my eyes for me. She couldn't see anything, however, through my left eye I saw things in the far left field of my vision as if I was seeing it though a fancy sort of crescent shape. That couldn't be right.

The next morning, I called for an appointment and on Thursday my ophthalmologist saw the problem -- a PVD, peripheral vitreous degeneration in each eye (more so in the left). To make a long story just a little longer, my boxing career came to an abrupt halt before it ever got started, but other than that I just get rechecked in about six weeks and probably will be all fine. (If a "curtain" like effect occurs in my field of vision, that would mean there is a retinal detachment and I would need to get to the doctor within 24 hours.)

What is great to me is that the doctor could see what I saw...and that means there was nothing to see in my brain. OK, that doesn't sound great. How about this? "There is nothing new in my brain that shouldn't be there."

All this week I have been thinking about Luke's account of the passion of Jesus. One of my favorite parts is Jesus' compassion toward the thief who is hanging on his own cross along side Jesus' cross. The thief says *"Jesus, remember me when you come into your kingdom."* Jesus responds, *"Truly I tell you, this day you will be with me in paradise."* What is that? Really? Jesus looks at someone who is really guilty and truly sees him...and loves him.

Vision. Seeing, through God-shaped-eyes. God knows there is dust on us, but knows the beauty underneath. And, even when our vision is distorted by dis-ease, God sees us through a lens of love -- the love that cannot be stopped by a cross or a tomb.

I am thankful to see....see new days....see the people whom I love.....but even more, I am thankful to be seen as you and the world are seen, with love, by God.

Butterflies and flowers
Posted Mar 30, 2013 7:42 p.m.

This last week I've received some lovely Easter cards from lovely people far and near....with designers named "Hallmark" and "Carlton" and such. Then one came, through another sister in Christ who, with others, had gone to visit men in the Dixon Correctional Facility for Bible Study, to do a simple craft project, and prayer. I made a similar trip a few years ago. This past week's project was to make Easter cards which they could send to their family members or friends. One man said that he wouldn't make a card. He had no one to send it to. He was assured that if he made a card, it would be sent to someone who would appreciate it. He did make a card. It came to me.The message is simple and true."Jesus love(s) you. Believe. Happy Easter."

So complicated. So simple.
Posted Apr 8, 2013 12:38 p.m.

"How do you feel?" "How's it going?" Just two of the sort of loving, simple questions that come my way pretty much each day from one person or another. Thank you, to the many of you who ask.

Here's the thing. When I know what the doctor says and what the scans say and what the lab reports report, I only know a fraction, a tiny fraction of how I "am." This last round of three-month-scans, now almost two months ago, proved that to me. Because of my re-worrying which re-started from the little re-growths of tumor in my right hip, I have spent an inordinately long time sorting out how I am. Certainly I like the "who I am" question so-so much better. (Laura = Child of God. Period.)

So, the truth is that the hip/tumor news was/is very distracting, particularly emotionally distracting. This is what has happened since.
1) About two weeks ago, I asked my counselor to go over the concept of "emotional memory" with me again. In short, this is the information I was looking for: Emotional memory can't "tell time." It has no sense of when

stuff happened. Emotional memory is always in the present. As a result, emotionally I can feel everything from the joy of the birth of my daughters to the grief of my husband's (or my) cancer diagnosis in no more than a second. I can "feel" them emotionally like they are happening right now. I can also "feel" the pain of anticipatory grief right now....like if I were to be more ill or to die soon and feel the pain of my parents or daughters or friends.

On the other hand, narrative memory is all about time. It knows and narrates our story. It knows things which happened 25 years ago or early this morning. It can tell the order of events. It knows I am not in the middle of something right now.

So, those two things are big deals to me. Those emotions of emotional memory of great events/fun stuff/joys and the like are emotions I love to relive and get energized about. This is not so much how I feel about the crappy stuff.

My counselor likens emotional memory to something like a big elephant, and narrative memory to something like a little person who is riding the big elephant and trying to guide the big elephant with no more than a stick. Emotions are powerful things.

So, this is where some of my centering prayer or meditation skills are helping.
 I have found that I cannot:
a) ignore emotional triggers.
b) repress my concerns/worries.
However, I can do this
I) - ask myself if I am safe NOW.
II) - ask myself if I am hurting/in pain/etc. NOW
III) - acknowledge the concern/worry/elephant and then let it walk on by.

Or, for those of you who like me use the image of leaves floating by on the stream in the creek that goes through the camp at LOMC (Lutheran Outdoor Ministry Center), just let that leaf (concern) float on by and go back to concentrating on that wonderful living water. This baptismal imagery is intended.

So, this helps me. It helps me a lot. It has helped me to explain to friends this "sorting out" that I do.
But, here's the thing....I still wonder how I'm doing. I haven't thought much about that because I was so very busy being a traffic director for elephants.
So....
2) I had a wonderful visit from a long time friend, who is also a wonderful writer. Within our conversation she mentioned a method called *The Writing Diet* by Julia Cameron. In short, Julia suggests that each day, early on, a person writes three lined 8 1/2 x 11 pages. No more. No less. She talks about how a person can lose weight by doing this.

I was more interested in how to lose burdens than weight. Now that I am a more practiced elephant traffic guide, I am more than ready to see what is going on inside of me. I am....alive. I am living. I am aching, and exercising anyway. I start crying sometimes and then I stop.

I love God and I love my family and friends. I plan stuff and then I do it. I do stuff that I haven't planned and enjoy that too. I highly suggest this.

April by the numbers
Posted Apr 13, 2013 6:26 p.m.

This morning I was reading the Gospel. Reading from John 21:1-19 that is assigned for tomorrow's (Sunday's) worship. It is the resurrection story of Jesus appearing to Peter and others as they were unsuccessfully fishing, when Jesus tells them to cast their nets on the other side of the boat and they make a huge haul: *So Simon Peter went aboard and hauled the net ashore, full of large fish, a hundred fifty-three of them; and though there were so many, the net was not torn.*
153: I love that. I say that somebody counted them. Somebody who found themselves overwhelmed by that blessing of fish....and every other amazing thing that Jesus did in those years. If ever I am feeling low, I can

usually turn that around by counting fish (a.k.a. blessings). Anyway, the whole thing got me thinking about numbers today, so here are some numbers for April:

4, then 3: Rabbits in the yard after I stood on the deck and chewed one of them out for using the tulip leaves as a salad bar, AGAIN.

50 plus: Number of daffodils that bloom in one bunch, in front of my house, in front of the dryer vent.

300: Number of dollars a new 3-person deck swing (with awning) was going to cost for the deck (on sale, free delivery, all assembly required).

63: Number of dollars the sale fabric cost me to recover the "vintage" deck swing and make a new awning for it.

30: Number of days until my next round of scans.

41: Number of pieces (squares, triangles, and one circle) which are sewn together to form EACH 12-inch square of the quilt I am starting for Erica. This thing had better be beautiful!

45: Approximate number of minutes it takes me to journal three college ruled pages "long hand" each morning.

2/3 yes, two-thirds: That is the amount of a one fish (probably a perch) that was "left" (a.k.a., FOUND BY ME) in the lawn shed in the back corner of my property. The only known sources of fish in my location are the Augustana Slough Pond, the Rock River, and the Mississippi River. I know that small animals tend to visit the shed, and I am guessing that the "aroma" in the shed is from something more than that petrified 2/3 end of a perch. It took a moment to compose myself, but I did manage to use a golf club swing weight trainer to extricate the perch from the shed floor and get on to the business of "fishing" the deck swing parts out of the shed (with Penny's help), so that the swing seat and awning could be measured, and fabric purchased...for $63, not $300.

Now that was only one fish, and not 153, so I'll count THAT as a blessing.

Got questions?
Posted Apr 15, 2013 9:59 a.m.

I have an iPhone 4S. Siri "lives" in it. It seems like she is willing to answer whatever question I give her, or to search the internet for the answer.

How many golfers are in the competitive field of the Master's?

Who won the Michigan vs. Louisville game?

What kinds of ornamental grasses are tolerant of any soil type and are 4-6 feet tall and are non-invasive?

Just because my phone CAN answer so many questions, that doesn't mean that "she" should be the only source for answers to my questions. In the last week, two young women whom I got to know via the Sarcoma Alliance group page on Facebook, went into hospice care. I looked to my iPhone for updates on Facebook this morning. There was one. Last night, one of them, Wendy Marie, mother of young Emma, died. For a while, I wished I hadn't even looked at my phone. I don't like all of the information it gives me.

I looked ahead to the readings for next Sunday. (John 10:22-30). I asked...what about these young women...what about me...what about all the people whose names I don't know but are suffering nonetheless?

I hear this in response....(John 10)

27 My sheep hear my voice. I know them, and they follow me.

28 I give them eternal life, and they will never perish. No one will snatch them out of my hand.

29 What my Father has given me is greater than all else, and no one can snatch it out of the Father's hand.

New shoes
Posted Apr 16, 2013 12:35 p.m.

The FedEx deliverer rang my doorbell and returned to his truck. A box containing new shoes sat on my front porch. I had just read on Facebook that people are wearing running/race shirts today to remember and honor the people who died or were injured in body/mind/spirit yesterday at the Boston Marathon.

Two weeks ago I realized that my hip pain may be worse because of the wear pattern of my walking shoes....the ones I have worn most days for the last year and a half. So I researched shoes. Tried stuff on. Shopped for the best deal. Ordered the color I liked. And, today they are here. I'm not a runner. If anything, I try not to run from stuff I need to deal with. Today though, I wear my new Saucony Cohesion 6 in blue/silver/citron, in love and remembrance. I have been thankful each day since my hip surgery that I still have my right leg and hip. Many people who have sarcoma require amputations to remove their tumors. So, for those who lose a limb to disease or disaster (in war time or in peace time), you have my prayers for healing and courage....and for what ever is needed for you to take the next step on the journey.

Pain, or "When it rains it pours"
Posted Apr 18, 2013 5:04 p.m.

This is a bit of an update, an update of the way I "felt" and what I did about it.

Last night, Wednesday, for about an hour and fifteen minutes or so, I had pain in the area of the pleural effusion in my left lung (lower, outer part of my left lung). It hurt when I breathed, not completely unlike the pain I had with pleurisy when I was 17-years-old. My creative mind moved a bit like my first car, a 1970-ish 2-door, V-8 Cutlass Supreme: zero to fast, quickly. I would be lying if I didn't say I was scared. Fortunately my lung felt better before I went to bed, and I slept all night. This morning it only gave an occasional twinge. However, my "scared" hadn't gone away. After some encouraging by a friend, I emailed Dr. Mo with what I had experienced.

Then I waited. While I waited, I wrote in my three-page-a-day journal....and checked my email about every two minutes. That is a rotten way to wait.

So, I tried this: I wondered what I wanted. I came up with "peace." Peace while I waited. I imagined a scene where Jesus gave that to his followers. The scene occurred during the time following Jesus' resurrection when he comes into the room where the disciples are locked up in fear and he breathes on them -- peace. I spent the better part of 20 to 30 minutes writing and imagining that peace....imagining Jesus' presence with the disciples and with me...giving over my worries and burdens....breathing, rather than holding my breath.

About two hours from my email delivery, I heard back from Dr. Mo with these instructions: If the pain is gone, then no worries. If it comes back and is constant/persistent/progressing, then it needs to be checked out, either locally or in Iowa City. Right now it is stable and non-painful.

So. I stay home and work on a project and wait for Erica to get home from work so she can shop-vac the water in the basement. Yep. There is water in the basement. Just in the usual places. Certainly, nothing like the flooding that other folks are having. It is still raining a bit so this will last a while. The thing is I know that some other folks are getting rained on right now -- some "actual rain" and some are getting poured on by "worry" or "pain" or "grief."

Some of them (you) are all locked up like the disciples, or me, last night. I am thankful for the peace that came while I was praying and writing. However, I also know when there is more going on than needs to be handled by prayer alone. Dr. Mo is also a gift from God.

"How am I?"
Posted Apr 24, 2013 11:37 p.m.

I am:
~ curious and joyful, because I have developed a 7-month class series entitled "Hope & Pray." We will study people in the Old and New Testament who have hoped and prayed for many things, such as healing, community, and children, and then look for connections in our own lives. Then we will try some new prayer practices. The planning alone makes me smile. I look forward to starting in May.
~ hopeful, because the lung pain, the bit of eye "blurriness," and the abdominal upset which I experienced last week are all gone this week.
~ proud, because of the good work Erica and Sarah are doing in work and school....and...
~ proud, because of the research and achievements which were celebrated in a Sigma Theta Tau (International Honor Society of Nursing), Theta Pi Chapter induction ceremony this last Sunday at IWU. I attended as a past president of this chapter and got to reconnect with former students and colleagues.

~ peaceful, probably because of our shared prayers. This comes as a bit of surprise, as the induction ceremony and the gathering which followed included reconnecting with people whom I had not seen -- some for 15-20 years. The fact that I remained peaceful, despite repeated telling of our family journey of these many years (including Rodney's death and my diagnosis), says something for your ongoing prayers and for the caring presence of the many nursing colleagues who were doing the asking.

~ excited, because I am just a week away from traveling to Ft. Lauderdale with my sister-in-law on our "Great (as in wonderful) Aunt Tour."

~ thankful, because of time with friends, feeling better, sunshine (even if it isn't warmer yet), both new hydrangea plants surviving the winter, worship in Bloomington last weekend

~ prayerful, because I can't think of another response to the frustration I feel for my friend Tanya and other Lutheran women called to ordained ministry in Australia, where ordination has been denied yet again.

~ much better than a year ago this time, because I year ago I was on chemotherapy, struggling with a very sick liver and all of the pain and worry that went with that therapy.

~ breathing and living each day, which is a good place to be at less than three weeks until my next scans.

Just right.
Posted May 3, 2013 5:15 p.m.

The sun is shining here in Fort Lauderdale. The breeze blowing. Lizards (no snakes) are sunning themselves. My sister-in-law, Dee, and I are enjoying the hospitality of Ben and Megan, our nephew and niece. Lunch in the tiki hut outside, followed by a leisurely private boat tour (by Megan) of the land and "floating" real-estate was wonderful. (We even got pictures alongside Johnny Depp's yacht!) I think this is just what Dr. Mo ordered. Living and loving life.

Things that help, Part 11
Posted May 10, 2013 10:40 a.m.

Today is my first full day at home in a week and a half. It is cool (50) and damp outside in Rock Island. (In comparison to sunny and 81 in Ft. Lauderdale. I think I need to take Ft. Lauderdale off my favorites on my iPhone....it isn't a fair comparison today!) I am looking outside rather than sitting under the shade of the tiki hut in my niece and nephew's back yard. However, the "message" I am getting here in Rock Island is still the same as the message last week in Florida.....and it is a "thing that helps." I am assailed by beauty and growing things. The blooming trees in my yard are spectacular. The one yellow tulip that survived the rabbit's pillaging is proud and tall. The grass is rich green and thick. The new palm tree that sprouted from a coconut as it floated in the river in Ft. Lauderdale, and traveled in a carry-on bag all the way to Illinois is comfortably set in a pot on the deck. In my view here, as in Ft. Lauderdale last week, every part of the earth that is not built on, or paved over is growing and blooming. And when I listen to it, I hear God saying "I love you. I love you all. Just look. I am healing you and soothing you and encouraging you and providing for you with the beauty of creation." It is "four sleeps" until my scans and appointments on Tuesday the 14th. I chose to listen to these words of encouragement and love from the Gardener.

Pondering....Mother's Day
Posted May 12, 2013 10:49 p.m.

Probably my favorite "mom story" in scripture is of Mary at the birth of Jesus. So much happened that day. Just having a baby "on the road" away from home would certainly be enough...then add to that the "accommodations in the stable, the early pregnancy angel visit, Joseph's decision to stick it out with her, ...and then this visit from those smelly ol' shepherds and their larger than life story of angels. It sounds like something that I would want to ponder in my heart for a while too! I wonder what her hopes were for her infant son in those first days. It has been my privilege to celebrate Mother's Days as a mom, myself, for 25 years. Today, honestly, I just wanted to have a meal with both of my daughters at home. I got my wish. It was great. Tomorrow, my folks will be here and I will get to share a meal with them on the "little-observed-day-after-Mother's-Day." That will be wonderful too.A big part of my coping and living on this journey is to practice the phrase "be here now." To focus on the present. To be thankful in the moment. Yet...I am now at less than 36 hours until I'm back in that MRI tube. It is time to look ahead too. (That is the reason my folks are coming tomorrow....they spend the night and we leave early on Tuesday morning for Iowa City.) So, this is what I'm pondering. I have even bigger wishes than a meal with my daughters and my Mom. I want good news on Tuesday. I want lots more meals. I want lots more Mother's Days. In fact, that's what I'm planning for. That's what I'm praying for; for me, for my family, for all y'all's families too.

Times for Tests on Tuesday
Posted May 13, 2013 9:19 p.m.

So, tomorrow goes like this....
6:45 a.m. -- Leave for Iowa City
8:10 a.m. -- Show up in MRI dept.
8:40 a.m. -- MRI scan
9:15 a.m. -- Dr. Buckwalter (the orthopedic surgeon) (I have no idea what time I will really end up seeing him, as that MRI and the related "stuff" takes more than 30 minutes).
12 noon -- Show up at CT department
12:30 p.m. -- CT scan (maybe without drinking the "yummy" grape drink because they are only scanning my lungs this time). Then.....LUNCH...I'll be hungry!
3:20 p.m. -- Dr. Mo (Dr. Mohammed Milhem, the oncologist) (This will likely start closer to 4:00 or so and can last 30 minutes some times...)
The traveling crew tomorrow includes my folks and daughter, Sarah.

Results for 5/14/13 Iowa City trip
Posted May 14, 2013 7:50 p.m.

1) You are some wonderful supporters and prayers. Truly I was peaceful through the whole day.
2) No chemo. That is good news in my book.
3) The hips tumors appear to be stable, although we are awaiting the final reading.
4) The lung tumors have grown but only very slightly. The larger tumors, only by 10-15% in size and the tiny ones by 50% or so, but these were only 1-2 mm to begin with.
5) So, I would prefer no growth; however, I am thankful for not having stuff going on that requires chemotherapy.
6) I am really looking forward to this summer with my daughters and family and friends.
7) It is good to be alive. It is good to live each day, acknowledging the gift from God.

Tornadoes and tests
Posted May 21, 2013 10:34 a.m.

This morning as the sun shone, the breeze blew, and the grass grew, the results came in. News stories and videos revealed that a horrible mile-wide tornado in Moore, Oklahoma devastated lives and homes and businesses. An email from Dr. Mo that my test results were in, revealed basically what he had said during my appointment last week....the tumors in my lungs are ever so slightly larger, one lymph node is a bit larger, the pleural space (where those effusions are) has tiny tumors (which was expected) and the right atrium of my heart might be a bit larger (which can happen when there is some sort of lung disease). One of the tumors in the operative area in my right hip has about .5 cm of enlargement, the rest remain the same.These are my conclusions: (1) None of this is a contest. I knew this already. All God's children have somethin' and all of us stand in need of God's grace. (2) People and relationships are way more important than stuff -- whether the stuff is what you live, work or go to school in, or what

243

is growing inside you. (3) The Lord is close to the broken hearted; and saves those who are crushed in spirit. Psalm 34:18. (4) I am and will continue to pray for those who were in the path of that tornado, and for the people who love them. And, I am going to go to my nephew William's high school graduation in New Albany, Mississippi with my folks, and then enjoy my extended Koppenhoefer family for the weekend.

Unlikely help...unlikely witness
Posted May 29, 2013 10:18 a.m.

This week the Gospel story from Luke tells of the faith of the Centurion -- of his belief that Jesus can heal his servant, even from a distance. And, Jesus does. In Hope & Pray, we studied the story from Daniel 3 of Shadrach, Meshach, and Abednego in the furnace of blazing fire, and of their deep faith....and that ol' King Nebuchadnezzar's surprising realization of the power of the One True God (a point that he has to re-learn several times). I figure that I am set for recognizing examples of faith and support in unlikely areas, and I have done so.

I have returned from a wonderful trip to Mississippi to witness a nephew's high school graduation, and also spent time with a Central Illinois family over a very wet Memorial Day Weekend. I returned home, to find my daughters faithfully caring for all the "stuff" in the basement, rescuing it from yet another basement-water-baptism.

And so I sit in the quiet of the morning, looking over my back yard with the Gospel reading, my journal and a cup of coffee. What do I see? A tree. An aging ornamental pear. It used to have a partner tree. The partner became diseased and died a few years ago. We are still trying to get grass to grow over that wound in the yard. This remaining tree has troubles of its own. It has a bit of the disease that the first tree had, and last year, it suffered a wound (from another falling tree) that took a big chunk out of its span on the North side. It has its own scars, too (from woodpeckers).

However, in due season, this remaining tree flowers beautifully and has put on a full crop of leaves as it reaches with ever growing branches toward the sun. Around its base, it puts out little tree shoots....trying to tell its tree story again and again. Yep. You probably guessed it. I'm a pastor with a lot of free time and many metaphors not-yet-spoken... recovering and living after the loss of my partner, living through disease and wounds and striving to grow and reach upward and keep blooming in due season. Like that tree, neither you nor I will live forever. However, we still have time to reach toward the Son and tell His story again and again.

"Me thinks she dost protest too much"
Posted Jun 5, 2013 10:17 a.m.

This morning, whilst journaling and reflecting on the events of the last day, I had a bit of an epiphany -- a lesson learned. I realized that there was something in me that made me not want to admit what I had learned. And, hence, that I had not really learned it. Here is some background information and what happened:

1) I really enjoy working in my yard. Plotting. Planting. Tending. In years past, a friend or family member would join in to help out with weeding or planting. The kids might mow or be coerced into trimming the hedge.

2) Two years ago, I really couldn't do much in the yard because of what I thought was sciatica. The last year and a half revealed another "s" word. Sarcoma.

3) In the time since that second "s" word was first announced in the doctor's office, I have done little to nothing in the yard. In this last month I've done some planting of pots for the deck and a bit of weeding. It has felt so good to do something -- anything! I also do some cheering of the current principal lawn care expert -- Erica. Last year, whilst in the midst of uncertain days and more pain, a few friends and a team of several families performed wonderful yard/garden work for us.

4) I went to read from the lessons for this next weekend. The First Lesson for this next Sunday is from 1st Kings (17:17-24) where Elijah, who has taken residence with the widow of Nain and her son, is confronted by the widow as her son has just taken ill and died. She calls on Elijah (if he really is a man of God) to do something besides just mooch off them.

245

Elijah takes the boy and has his own grown-up-conversation with God -- facing his own doubts, pleads to God, and the boy lives.

5) So what is that about? Is it just that God is the real deal? That even "famous people/prophets" have doubts? That bad stuff happens to good people? That suffering is universal? These are all certainly true.

6) Today...for me....one point is that the widow asked for help. Real help. The "he's dead and there is no other hope" kind of in your face "you do something" kind of help. -- But no! I looked back at it again. She doesn't ask for help. She just gets mad at God and at Elijah. I thought she asked for help she didn't. Does that matter? Does that matter to God? This story isn't just about the widow and the son and God....it is about Elijah too. This situation provided an opportunity for him to get himself square with God, for him to pour out his doubts and hopes and trust to God, and even see God's power returned as a blessing to the woman and her son.

7) I can imagine the widow's joy. Her son is alive. Today, I can also imagine the joy of Elijah as he was able to offer God's help to someone else.

8) Here's the deal. Because I can do a little bit, I haven't asked for help. It is like I turned on a "personal control and self sufficiency" switch. And...I have been happy to do so! I have equated being healthy with being able to "do it all" for myself. Even though I am not as well as I want to be, I have pretended by just turning on the darn switch. It turns out that there are friends and family that want to help -- not just when I feel lousy, but when I feel better too!

9) Why is this lesson something I have to keep learning? Life is meant to be lived in community. There are "Elijahs" all over the place who are ready and willing and actually wanting to be asked to help. They want to see how God will work through them. They want some of that joy as well.

10) (which is plenty...) I want to remember that when I ask for help it doesn't mean that I am standing on my last leg, or that I have failed, or that God has failed me, or that the end is near....it just means that life is better lived when we all stand together.

Compassion, and what makes a difference
Posted Jun 8, 2013 11:01 a.m.

This morning, with the sun shining on the yard, the flowers growing and blooming, I read again from Luke of Jesus' compassion for the widow whose son had died....and he raised him. The gospel commentary writer reminded me that Luke used the word "Lord" for Jesus in that story, rather than the name Jesus. He suggested that what it means to be Lord isn't to be some far off ruler. It is to be with people. To see their struggles first hand, have compassion, and heal. This isn't a picture of some "far away God" or some "looks good on paper" or a "Hey, I made you...good luck with your life!" sort of God. This is an "I'm with you every step of the way" God. This is really important to me.

Last night, friends gathered at our home to celebrate our friend Penny's completion of the Northern Illinois Synod's Diakonia study. It was a lovely evening. Great friends. Great food. Beautiful yard (thanks to Erica and Penny's hard work). The evening grew cooler and I distributed some of my prayer shawls and quilts to those who were cool in the early June air. (One beautiful shawl arrived just this week....) Then I put on a pot of water for several to have cups of hot tea. June. Go figure.

The talking shifted to caring conversations about people we know who are or have recently struggled with cancer. The dear friend of one person had died that day. When she said that that person didn't have the experience of mat-carriers, and prayers, and prayer shawls.... She said she could see that those things truly made a difference for me. That my faith makes a difference for me. It does. I said that I don't know if it is adding to the quantity of my days, but I am confident that it adds to their quality.

Joy and grief and prayers.
Posted Jun 13, 2013 9:41a.m.

In keeping with my desire/attempt/striving to ask for help when I need it....here it goes.

Joy. Our synod assembly begins tomorrow morning. It is held at Augustana College in Rock Island -- just a few blocks from my house.

247

This year is the 10th Anniversary of my ordination. I have always loved synod assembly. The worship, the Bible study, the introducing parishioners to this beautiful expression of the church, seeing colleagues. (Last year I didn't go because I was still suffering the effects of the chemotherapy and still couldn't walk well).

Grief. This year I have really wanted to go to some of the assembly. However, this morning I am just in a puddle about it. As I get closer to it, the thought of being there seems to enumerate so many of my losses and then stands them up in front of me....and I weep. ....I don't want to go if I am just going to cry through the whole thing. Yet, I truly know that God is in that place, in that worship, in those people gathered...and I want to be there as well.

What I'm learning - Part 1
Posted Jun 15, 2013 8:46 a.m.

It is a rainy morning, the second day of synod assembly. Yesterday morning I provided the "watering." Maybe today it is the sky's turn. In brief....this is what I learned so far:

~ Asking for help makes a difference. It puts me in better relationship with God, with myself, and with others. When I ask for help, I can then look for that help to come, and it has. Certainly being reunited with treasured friends and colleagues was emotional for me, yesterday. However, the tears revealed more than my griefs. It also revealed my deep caring for them and for the ministry we share.

~ We needed to see each other. I had thought that I just needed to see "them." After all, I missed "them." I really hadn't realized the importance of the "them" seeing me.

What I am learning - Part 2 "One"
Posted Jun 21, 2013 10:29 a.m.

"One" I knew this before I went to synod assembly, which was almost a week ago now. I still know it...but I know it even deeper in my bones. It is all about "One."

248

"One" Years ago, while on internship, I went to visit a home bound church member. She was struggling because she wasn't able to come to worship any more. She wasn't able to volunteer as she used to. Then she told me of her prayers for the folks on the prayer chain, though she never saw them. Then she told me of how she gave the Children's Bulletin, which she received with the Sunday worship bulletin, to her housekeeper's child, and talked to her about Jesus. While she grieved the ministry she missed, I affirmed the ministries she had. She prayed. She told the story. That was beautiful. That was the shape of her ministry at that stage in her life.

"One" For almost two years, there were folks whom I knew through ministry settings, whom I didn't get to see at all. However, I knew they were praying for me. There were countless times when, though I was physically alone (at home, or in an MRI tube, or wherever, I was worried), that I had peace, knowing I was lifted up in prayer and loving thoughts of so many.

"One" I take you to John 17. Chapter 13 begins the Last Supper.....and Jesus' long discourse with the disciples after he washes their feet and tells them to love one another. As Chapter 18 begins, Jesus goes to the garden to pray and is arrested and continues his journey to the cross and resurrection. Chapter 17 is a bit of a tricky read. It goes long and seems to loop over and back, with lots of repeats, but it is worth the read. It is Jesus. Praying for his disciples "and all who will believe" because of the disciple's word -- that "they may all be ONE." How about that? We all, as in us and them, and those, and people we don't even know, and people we haven't even lived in the same century with, and people yet to come-- have been included in this prayer.

"One" When I pray, I imagine myself and the one for whom I pray all held close to Christ....so close....so close in fact that we are one. Not one as in "agreeing" on everything. Not one as in "the same." But, one as in "in one loving relationship together, where each of us bring our best selves." In that relationship, there is no brokenness for all are whole and well.

"But I'm not prepared for that!"

Posted Jul 1, 2013 9:42 a.m.

Last week, on early Tuesday morning, I sat down with the lectionary readings for this past Sunday, and wrote my sermon for First Lutheran Church in Rock Island, where I presided and preached for Pastor Mayer as he traveled in Sweden and Norway. Having that sermon written early made for a wonderful week.

Then Saturday came. I figured I would pull out that sermon and tweak it a bit. Done. Then I pulled out that bulletin rough draft that had been printed for me to review the liturgy. All was well until I got to the readings; they didn't match the ones I had used to prepare! Oh. My. Goodness! I looked high and low in every resource to figure out who had the "correct texts" and where the ones in the draft bulletin had come from. The only time I could find that particular text in the rough draft bulletin assigned for use was to look ahead to 2016! (These are the things that pastor's nightmares are made of! Staying calm (not really, but let's pretend I was), I drove over to the church (in the pouring rain -- for real, not just for dramatic effect), and found that stack of freshly prepared bulletins for the following day -- Whew. The texts were "right." My sermon could stand as prepared. Sunday went just fine.

The folks of First Lutheran in Rock Island are gracious people. It was an honor to lead their worship.

However....I've been thinking about that brief bit of terror that came over me; the "but I'm not prepared for THAT!" for the past 48 hours. In those hours I've done a number of things "for the first time;" like yesterday, to try to track down church organists for a possible funeral at a church where I am not a member, and this morning, to figure out how to clean up my beautiful deck bench after my local raccoon used it as a toilet. I guess the point is that I (we) do stuff every day that we don't think we are prepared for.

This morning, I read the gospel for next Sunday (even though I am not preaching in worship). It is about Jesus sending out the 70, two by two, ahead of him... to prepare the way --- cure people and announce that the Kingdom of God has come near. I'm guessing they weren't feeling 100% prepared. I'm figuring that a seminary degree, years of pastoring and a lifetime of worshipping and loving God, life in a community of faithful, seeking, Spirit-filled people, and the Spirit's calling are plenty to have me prepared. But, am I prepared for this?....

This month of July is Sarcoma Awareness Month. Honestly, before two years ago, I'm not even sure I was aware of sarcoma as much more than on a list of other cancers. I have spent some part of my life encouraging people to have a colonoscopy (after Rod's cancer), to have mammograms (after my Grandma Davis', and numerous friends' cancers), to stop smoking (after my father-in-law's cancer) and to use sunscreen (after melanoma diagnosis in my extended family). Now it is "Sarcoma Month." That is an odd thing to think after every month since September of 2011 has been sarcoma month for me. It would be nice if there was an "early" way to detect sarcoma. There are so very many types of sarcomas that is hard to even say where to start looking...and by the time they are found, they can do quite a bit of damage, and most often, move on, likely to the lungs as in my case.

Precious
Posted Jul 6, 2013 9:32 a.m.

I'm not quite sure why, but the word "precious" has been stuck in my head for several days...and that's a good thing. I've even been singing "precious" ("Jesus loves the little children..."). I went to a Bible search program on the computer and found "precious," referred to many times as something "as precious as" jewels or stones, or silver or gold, or ointment or oil, or faith. It made me think about why I considered what I had been doing or seeing as precious. So....here is a view through my eyes of what precious things surround me, or I have coming up:

1) Pictures of our family Fourth of July celebrations over the years... decorated strollers and bicycles, flags flying, smiling faces....and this year's photo with my daughters.

2) Time in crop surveys....in my mom's flower garden...in my own flower gardens....in my father's fields... In seeing what "second year" hydrangeas and Amazing Grace day lilies are doing.

251

3) The voices of the children at First Lutheran in Rock Island as we explored Jesus' love for us with his "face set toward Jerusalem" as parents taking their hurting child to the emergency room to be healed.

4) Preparation for a "Quilt Garden Tour" with Mom next week to Elkhart, Indiana....and a vacation in Mississippi to follow that.

5) The realization that my back pain is lessening.

6) Long summer days with no chemotherapy.

7) The voices of my family in prayer before meals.

8) Time spent caring for friends....plotting with friends.....playing with friends.....crying with friends.....laughing with friends.

9) Thoughts of hope....writing HOPE in the sand at the beach...and suggesting to fellow sarcoma survivors on a sarcoma Facebook site, that though hope may be washed away, we can rewrite it anew each day....

10) Quiet mornings....in prayer, in hope, in the bright sun and cool breeze, on the journey...A good neighbor.

A Good Neighbor
Posted Jul 12, 2013 4:58 p.m.

I was thinking this afternoon about that Good Samaritan story...about who is my neighbor and such. Today I am in Pontiac, Illinois, resting up between trips. Mom and I returned from a bus trip with the McLean County Chapter of the University of Illinois Home Extension Master Gardeners to explore the Quilt Gardens of Elkhart County, Indiana. Tomorrow, we leave for Mississippi for several days. So, for a minute, I pause to say thanks for my home town, Pontiac.

Last night we went to a Vermillion Players children's production of *The Little Mermaid, Jr.* which was wonderful. Tonight we will hear the Pontiac Municipal Band play their weekly Friday evening outdoor concert; these are a musical gift. Besides "blowing a horn" for my home town (which has done a remarkable job with its downtown, and tourism, and the arts) it is the people of Pontiac that I extend my thanks to. Each place I go, I encounter yet another person who has held me and my family in prayer. That, my neighbor, is a gift beyond measure.

Pie tins, curling ribbon, and putting it all together
Posted Jul 20, 2013 9:46pm

I am a determined person. This year, among other things, I have been determined to grow sunflowers. Again. Last year, friends had to dig and fence and plant my sunflower plot, but by golly those sunflowers grew. This year, I still needed help with the digging, planting, and fencing, but when 97% of the sunflowers became seed for the local birds, the plot had to be replanted.

This time, however, I tried my own "secret weapon" which I was sure would scare off any birds. I cut up wedges of pie tins and strung them up in pairs with yellow curling ribbon and hung them from wire stakes at varying heights within the "sunflower playpen." When the wind blows, the tins "jingle" (...in an incredibly terrifying way, of course). Yes, sure, my family and friends were ready to nominate me for redneck of the year, but hey, I'm determined.

Then I left for two weeks. Erica and Penny watered the garden while I was gone. And, "ta-da!," now I have sunflowers growing. I'm home now, and watering those sunflowers myself. And, as I stood soaking the ground this evening, I had another thought or two about my determination. It seems like down deep I really wanted those sunflowers....a sign of hope for people with sarcoma, and a remembrance of fun and gardens-past for my family, to be there; to stick around. Part of me would move heaven and earth (or cut pie tins and string curling ribbon) to keep hope alive.

Or, was that even it? Was it really about hope? I think what I would REALLY like to do is to put a fence around my daughters, my family, my friends, and dangle those tins to keep away ANYthing that would rob them of joy and life and hope. However, I can't.

Tonight, I remembered this....still full from a delicious meal at Johnny's Steak House with my daughters, celebrating Rod's and my 28th wedding anniversary. It was delicious and the time spent with my daughters is cherished, but that isn't how anniversaries are supposed to be spent. Not with your kids; just with your spouse. I grieve that we didn't have a fence tall enough or pie tins big enough to keep cancer from Rod....or from me. I am not going to be able to protect my flowers from whatever will happen in life....let alone fence in my kids or the rest of the people I care about.

"Free will" is a gift I hold very precious as well. And, "accepting" cancer, or what ever is the marauder-of-the-day, isn't an easy or even desirable direction to go. However, what I do choose to do in the midst of whatever comes each day is love. I am ever so thankful to be loved as well....by God and by so very many people.

Jesus responded time and time again to the disciples that all they were called to do, all they were asked to do, was to love God and love one another. He was right on. That IS something within my capacity to do. Every day. Most of the time we really don't know "why our friend/spouse/child/neighbor has cancer/mental illness/arthritis/dementia."

Most of the time when we ask "why" it is because we don't want it to happen to ourselves. (Prevention IS good, after all.) However, what we do want to know is what we can do about it. It is this: Love. Whatever that looks like to you. To me. To our neighbor.

Muscles.
Posted Aug 2, 2013 10:42 a.m.

I've been doing some thinking about "muscles" lately....

1) "Quilting muscles:" I am going to need them, as it is time to do the "quilting" on the quilt that I've made for Sarah. I have two weeks to get this done before she goes back to college. I think I can....I think I can.

2) "Physical/actual muscles:" I have been pretty achy lately (OK, for a long time, but....) but I have not done any of my exercising since I messed up my back with that sunflower planting "incident" when I'd decided to plant the area myself rather than waiting for help. So, I am gradually reintroducing exercise. So far, it is helping me sleep better, and my right hip has some focal areas of sharp pain. So, this is all about balance.

3) "Spiritual muscles:" recently I led a book discussion group on the third book in *The Walk* series by Richard Paul Evans. I am currently reading book #1 and have read #3 and #4. Each of them can work as stand-alone-books, but the longer story is of a man who "had it all" as an advertising executive with a beautiful, smart wife. His wife dies from an infection after a horseback riding accident paralyzed her. His partner steals his business, and his house and cars are repossessed. So, he goes on a "walk"

from Seattle to Key West, Florida. He encounters some fascinating people along the way and learns quite a bit. At some point he is also diagnosed with a brain tumor. While I share some life experiences with this character (Alan), and certainly some emotional experiences as well, I have a much more rich and strong base of my faith, family, and friends.

Though my family and friend relationships have strengthened in recent years, however, I feel these were always present. My spiritual muscles have been present, and tested and strengthened too. I guess I mention the spiritual muscles because I know that I draw on that strength every day...recently on behalf of several friends' families and my own extended family during their experiences of cancer diagnoses and/or surgeries. The great thing about spiritual strength is not so much that I (or you) am strong, but that Christ is. Frankly, some of my experiences of late have taken me to the ground, with no place to go but up. I wish I didn't know this (because it is knowledge born of trial), but God's help in those times has been beyond my imagining, and I am thankful.

Putting the pieces together
Posted Aug 9, 2013 10:37 a.m.

The sun is shining. The humming bird has already dined on the flowers on the deck. I check out the readings again for Sunday, and I laugh. (Matt. 6)
Make purses for yourselves that do not wear out, an unfailing treasure in heaven, where no thief comes near and no moth destroys.
I have made no purse, but rather the first of two quilts; this one for Sarah, the next one for Erica. The material is actually some of Rod's clothing; many yellow golf shirts, some jeans, some khaki pants, and oxford cloth dress shirts stored in the basement in Rubbermaid Totes for the past 8 1/2 years, where no moth would destroy them.
I get the Gospel writer's point -- don't count on your "stuff" and love it above God, or it becomes your love and your god. (*For, where your treasure is, there your heart will be also.*)
Putting those pieces together for the quilt over the past few weeks has been a sort of treasure, though. While I was concerned that the project

would be too big, or too hard, or too taxing, or some other sort of "too", it has actually been good, and healing....and a gift of love.

This week I am thinking of two other "quilts" of sorts....one is the quilt I will make for Erica out of some other stuff from that tote. I will start that in another month or so, after we celebrate her 25th birthday.

The other "quilt" is one that Dr. Mo is working on, as am I. My next scan is a little less than a month away on September 3. I learned this week of a new clinical trial of a sarcoma drug that is actually offered locally. This morning I checked the National Cancer Institute site of the National Institute of Health, on their Clinical Trials page. It turns out that that a new chemo drug (Alisertib) is offered at Iowa City as well, and Dr. Mo is the lead investigator on that study there. It works by blocking an enzyme that makes cells grow. The goals of the study are to determine the response rate of various sarcomas to the drug, and to calculate the PFS (progression free survival) and OS (overall survival) of people on the medication.....oh yes, and to figure out what the side effects are.

I imagine what Dr. Mo does is examine each drug and each treatment, to see what is best, most lovely, most fitting for each person, and pieces together what is just right for a particular time and need. I don't usually head to the internet much anymore regarding sarcoma, except to see that there continue to be new medicines there for trial to combat the 70 or more types. (I think I have heard from only one person who has been on this study.) Too much internet "travel" keeps me from seeing the beauty that is around me right now!

There is an art to assembling each of these kinds of quilts. There is beauty and the potential for healing in all of them. However lovely they are, I am reminded that my truest treasure is God's gift of grace beyond measure.

Location, location, location
Posted Aug 14, 2013 11:17 a.m.

Today, as most days, "it is all about location."

1) Today's "location to be re-purposed" at home is the main floor sunroom. Currently the part-office, part-plant-nursery, part-quilt-factory, will temporarily be the place-to-put-the-stuff-Sarah-is-taking-to-her-college-apartment. This is only temporary. She leaves on Saturday (August 17). Then, of course, a part of my heart will have a temporary location in Normal, Illinois once again....and so it goes.

2) My location this morning had been with-coffee-at-the-dining-room-table-watching-hummingbirds. At the same time I was watching the ELCA Church Wide Assembly in Pittsburg, PA, livestreaming feed on my computer. I tuned in, just as four of the candidates for presiding bishop were answering questions and a vote was taken. Now it stands that two of the three remaining candidates (one being Presiding Bishop Mark Hanson) are women. I am thankful for the opportunity to "be present" from my location. I am thankful to sing and pray with them through this time. I am also thinking of my brothers and sisters in the Lutheran Church in Australia, who pray, work, and dream to have a day when women can be ordained pastors, and bishops, and presiding bishops.

3) And lastly, about a "change of location." The brothers and sisters of the three Rock Island Lutheran Churches, where I have enjoyed teaching in this past nine months are hosting a 10th Anniversary of Ordination reception for me. The date is Sunday, August 18 from 2-4 p.m.

The LOCATION has changed. The new location is St. James Lutheran Church at 3145 31st Ave.

Why has it changed? Months ago, when the date and location were selected, it seemed that the new parish hall addition at St. John's would be completed easily by this time. It is so close to being done....but not quite! In the grand scheme of things it is *much* more important that the building be finished well -- as it is truly a gift of the congregation in outreach to the community. The St. James community is gracious to offer their wonderful space for this celebration, and I am thankful.

By the numbers...

Posted Aug 21, 2013 1:43 p.m.

1... Daughter (Sarah) moved into her apartment at Illinois State last Saturday

2... projects; one knitting and one crocheting are ready for some work this week as I travel. I am not the driver.

3... third trip of stuff being delivered to ISU today (One- she did ahead, Two - with her when she started living there last Saturday, Three - today....the last little stuff....suits, calculator, etc.)

8...approximate number of hours it will take for my brother-in-law, Rick, to drive Dee and me to Tennessee for a 4-day Cousins' Reunion starting tomorrow.

13...more days until my next round of scans on Tuesday, September 3 in Iowa City (prayers, as always, welcomed).

150... springerle cookies....either anise flavored or cran-raspberry flavored, are ready for taking to the reunion!

Countless!... The thanks I offer to the many, many people who helped to prepare for, host, and attend the Ordination Anniversary Reception. It was a wonderful afternoon, and after 24 hours, I was feeling rested and ready to go again!

$600...amount of money donated at, or around the time of the reception, for the ELCA and Lutheran World Relief Anti-Malaria Campaign.

This means that 60 households can use mosquito nets to protect their family members from mosquito borne malaria each night as they sleep.

Back on the mat. Carry on.

Posted Aug 29, 2013 9:40 a.m.

Even people with a graduate degree in nursing, and a graduate degree in ministry, people like me (actually me) don't take their own advice or direction well. Yep. Guilty. So, when I returned from the cousins' reunion in Tennessee....and noticed a little rash on my abdomen, and watched it for about 24 hours, and noticed it got worse, and blistered and started to burn, even I decided to talk to a few doctors. First I talked to my brother, the doctor, and then I talked to Dr. Mo. Perhaps....perhaps it was shingles. That wouldn't be good. So, I started on an antiviral medication. Then, the next day, as I sat on the exam table, examined by my nurse practitioner, the little secret that I had kept for about two weeks, that I had experienced some chest pain came pouring out of me. My, oh, my, I had not wanted to get back on that mat and be carried around, even if it were to be carried by you dear people to see if Jesus had any healing tricks up his sleeve, by way of his local "hands and feet." (a.k.a. my health care team)

After my confession, an EKG revealed a normal rhythm. After I talked with Dr. Mo, he agreed that it would be just fine (as the nurse practitioner suggested) to get a cardiac stress test. (Just to be sure I am fine.) Perhaps, the ultimate irony -- or ultimate working of the Spirit -- or both, was that this week was the week during which I lead the "Hope & Pray" groups....and the text that I had chosen 5 months ago for this week was (you guessed it --) Mark 2:1-12, the story of Jesus healing the paralyzed man, who had been carried by his friends to Jesus. Yep. I was "paralyzed."

Sometimes it seems just too much to imagine or accept that another thing could go wrong. I was stuck, going nowhere, until I asked for help, and accepted the help that was given. So....what steps are next on this journey? (1) Forgiving myself for not speaking up when I first experienced that ol' chest pain. (2) Remembering that just because my family is in the middle of transitions I still need to care of myself. (3) Accept your mat carrying and prayers for my cardiac stress test tomorrow (Friday, August 29) and my next quarterly scans on Tuesday, September 3. (I will get the results for all of the tests on Tuesday). (4) Accept your prayers for the healing of my tummy....that this is either not shingles....or is responding to the medication. (5) Prayers for courage and wisdom are welcomed as well.

Here's an idea...
Posted Aug 30, 2013 6:56 p.m.

Here's an idea: Let's "induce" something OTHER than stress.I can come up with a whole list... Really! For instance:
Joy.

Hope.
Laughter.
Humor.
Deliciousness.
Fun.
Compassion.
Curiosity.
You get the idea.
Cardiac stress tests induce, you guessed it, stress. This sort of stress is like a combination of the worst migraine ever, plus all of the hot-flashes ever, plus all of the nausea from morning sickness ever, plus running a marathon while lying down, plus shortness of breath --- all happening within about two minutes from the "giving" of the "medicine" to induce "stress."
I guess that they also induced "thankfulness" for the following things:
1) that I did not have chest pain at all during the three and a half hours or so that I was there having a variety of scans
2) that the techs and nurses were wonderful
3) that I am in fact done with the hot flash portion of my life
4) that I received the "antidote" medicine for the "stress" and it worked
5) that a dear friend accompanied me and kept me smiling and laughing while I waited between tests
6) that the nausea that I am currently still feeling is related to having to take my regular meds without the benefit of food in my stomach and will at some point go away
7) that I had SO many prayers during that whole experience.

For everything there is a season; Scan Time
Posted Sep 2, 2013 9:38 p.m.

Yep....for everything there is a season ....(*Turn. Turn. Turn.*...by the Byrds....) Or....Ecclesiastes 3....
Today has been a "season" for painting the front porch (Mom and Dad), and spreading mulch (Erica, Mom and Dad).
Tomorrow (Tuesday, September 3) is the "season for scans." So, my dear supporters and pray-ers (Mat carriers)...here is the schedule:

7:15 a.m. Leave for Iowa (FYI....I have to "stop" eating at 4:45 a.m.)
8:45 a.m. CT scan of lungs/chest.
10 a.m. MRI scan of hips/pelvis.
11 a.m. Dr. Buckwalter.
1:20 p.m. Dr. Mo.
Update....no further chest pain....no more rash.

And the results are in...
Posted Sep 3, 2013 5:00 p.m.

The tumors are all still growing, slow and steady. Maybe there are a few new ones. We debated chemotherapy and Dr. Mo went through the various types. In short, I decided to wait to start chemo. We re-evaluate in December.

Lost "in"
Posted Sep 12, 2013 3:42 p.m.

Since returning from Iowa City last week, I've found that I am most comfortable getting "lost in" things....for instance:
~ the preparations for Erica's 25th Birthday Celebration last
Saturday...which was a wonderful day...and fun days preceding it as well.
Although her actual birthday is October 11, we opted for a celebration
when the yard was still in full bloom.
~ the clear warm water of the fitness center swimming pool....trying to do
an exercise that "buffers" the effort on the hip, yet moves some air into my
lungs. (I am trying to keep that air moving, as there is an area of lung
compression which is a bit larger than the last time I was scanned).
~ some little crocheting projects...fun, simple, pretty....
~ going through the monthly bills/receipts/Quicken updates (OK...it is
possible to do a bit too much of this.)
It seems like when I poke my head up from my "lost location," everything
is still there....the wondering about when chemo might start, about what
the cardiologist will say when I meet with him tomorrow about some
"artifact" in my stress test.

261

The Gospel lesson this week includes two of Jesus' parables about "lost stuff" (Luke 15:1-10)....a sheep and a coin, and the joy of finding them. I truly know that Jesus is in whatever place I am choosing to lose myself at that moment. This morning on the swing on the deck, I meditated as I was watching the hummingbirds and cardinals make their morning rounds. I imagined myself burrowed into a big blanket on Jesus' lap....occasionally peeking out to see where I was, deciding I was quite comfortable there, and returning to my original position. It's nice here for a while. Jesus has tissues.

Maybe yes, maybe no
Posted Sep 13, 2013 6:58 p.m.

It is hard to take a good picture of a heart....I mean an actual heart. It keeps beating. It is surrounded with bones and tissues. I have always thought I was good-hearted. Or, at the very least, I most always mean well. But this heart thing, as in my actual one, is a tough thing to "pin down." So, this is what I know:
1) I have not had a heart attack.
2) I did fine with the stress part of my stress test.
3) There is some sort of artifact that makes it look like I have a scar on the front (anterior) part of my heart....
4) My shortness of breath has to do with the pleural effusions.
5) The chest pain is not a normal thing to have.
6) I could have 1-2 tests to get a better picture of what is going on with my heart (an echocardiogram and a heart CT).
7) At this point, I am thinking that I will probably have both tests, because of the likelihood of having chemotherapy.
8) It could be that my first chemo was a little hard on my heart (although I didn't have this problem when I was actually on the chemo).
9) I'm going to check in with Dr. Mo and talk it through with him.
10) I do like Dr. Puri, the cardiologist, whom I saw today at Cardiovascular Medicine (CVM) in Moline.
11) Your prayers "warmed my heart."

Getting tackled, or not
Posted Sep 23, 2013 11:23 a.m.

It's fall. I have only seen a bit of football in person -- Rocky taking on Quincy last week; watching the game until the marching band performed the half time show. Then, I was homeward bound. Other than that, about all I know is that the Bears are 3-0 and my great niece has been loving playing jr. high football in Leroy, Illinos, and her brother has been loving playing football in high school, too. My niece has just been tackled by whatever virus is going around. Somehow something clobbered me too. If this is how football season is, I don't like it. I am a pretty careful study of my usual aches, and realized that the current stuff is new.

So, yesterday afternoon, I made the decision to admit that it had knocked me out of my position in the starting line up for the Professional Leaders Conference, which I planned to attend for the first day and a half. I have missed the last two years and really wanted to be there this year. The little sore throat and aches haven't completely knocked me out, but they have certainly sidelined me.

1) I am hoping to return to water exercise when I feel better....get this -- because it made me feel better! I have been doing this regularly for two weeks and REALLY hope that this field of play isn't the source of my cold.

2) Dr. Mo would like me to have the heart tests....the first is this Friday (echocardiogram) and the second (heart CT) is awaiting insurance approval, which may or may not come.

3) Erica and I have started on her quilt. I am glad for this....for the time with her and the beauty of what we are creating.

4) This morning I read the story of Lazarus and the rich man (Luke 16:19-31) which is the Gospel for this next Sunday. I have to admit that the feeling of being "tormented," even by little, ongoing aches and/or worries, could get the best of me. What am I saying? Some days it does get the best of me. However, perhaps the best defense is a good offense. So, in my journalling today I came up with 25 things I could do INSTEAD of sitting and hurting/worrying. It wasn't even hard to come up with 25. I could have gone on, but I had reached my page limit. For now, it is time to get back in the game. I think I'll thank the Coach, and then hit the showers.

Just a tiny bit...
Posted Sep 30, 2013 11:06 a.m.

This morning I looked ahead to the Gospel for next Sunday (Luke 17:5-10). I see a bunch of overwhelmed disciples. They are trying to figure out how to live out all that Jesus has proposed for them. Wow. They take deep breaths. They sigh. They ask, "Increase our faith!" That makes some sense to me. They could have asked for better walking shoes with arch support. Or a Platinum Master Card to cover their expenses on the road. Or a Torah app for their smart phones. What is so wrong with asking for more faith?
Jesus says-- *"If you had faith the size of a mustard seed, you could say to this mulberry tree, 'Be uprooted and planted in the sea,' and it would obey you."*
I like the seed imagery. Most of the time. I look out at my yard and see a table full of fancy gourds and some pumpkins that grew from just a few seeds. In fact, I see a whole bunch of things still blooming which came from tiny seeds. I even carry a mustard seed (laminated in clear packing tape) in my billfold in my purse...just to remind me of this particular story in scripture, and of Jesus' words. The thing is, I also know that just a teeny tiny bit of a cancer cell can also cause a whole lot of trouble. Last week when I had that echocardiogram, I think my heart looked just lovely if I do say so myself. However, it was trickier to get to see because of the fluid between the two pleural layers around my left lung (the pleural effusion) which is there because of some tiny little "seed." It seems that I probably won't have the results of that test until some time after October 7.
Yet. I know two other things:
1) Those tiny little cancer cells have also resulted in me receiving the overwhelming love, care and support of countless people.
2) Jesus is right. It isn't all about the amount of my/our faith....it is about the One in whom we have faith.

A reason for thanks...
Posted Oct 4, 2013 11:40 a.m.

In the last few days I've had an off-and-on relationship with the blues again. It seems that I am still able to ignore some of the lovely breezes of the Spirit, blowing delightful things gently through my life. Then, one afternoon this week, I got a phone call from the college-student-daughter of a long time friend. She offered me a special gift. As a part of a project for class, she was to write someone a letter of thanks, for what that person has meant in their life. Then she was assigned to contact that person and read them the letter. I was that person. What a powerful experience! It was as if the Holy Spirit attached herself to a blower and pointed it right at me! She mentioned that they learned how gratitude increases happiness. I know that she increased both in me.

Persistence
Posted Oct 17, 2013 10:57 a.m.

I've been thinking about persistence for a few days now. I read about other people who have similar diagnoses, and how they have had a hard time getting accurate diagnoses....and how much persistence it takes to get good care.

I watch a ground hog coming through my yard and how he/she enjoys the Black Eyed Susans, even returning for more on the day after I have chased him/her away with my most menacing "Hey! Move on!" shouted from the deck.

I have been putting little missives about my pleural effusions and my labored breathing (on exertion) in God's in-box several times a day. I guess that if they are going to persist, then I will persist in making them someone else's (God's) problem too. I know that I can talk to Dr. Mo if they trouble me more.

Then, Monday, I did my scripture study on the Gospel for Sunday, and a little light gardening. It turns out, I'm not the only persistent one. In the story from Luke 18, Jesus tells the parable of the "persistent widow" who keeps pleading her case to the judge, until the judge gives in and grants her case because of her persistence....not necessarily based on the validity of the claim (we just don't know about that). Many times this text is used to encourage us to be persistent in prayer....because God hears us.....because God heard "even the widow"....right? (As a widow of almost nine years, I will tell you that it seems like every other story seems to be about widows, but that is a story for another day.) Anyway. Another friend, Rev. Janet Hunt tells the story of teaching a class using this text. One of the students in a class she was leading in a seminary pondered "What if the 'widow' is Jesus, who is persistently pleading to God on our behalf?" Wow! I think so...

If the widow is me or you, then the argument that (1) if you plead long and hard enough then, (2) you will get what you want and (3) if you don't then (4) you didn't ask enough is baloney!

Perhaps even a better picture for me is the Spirit *interceding for us, with sighs to deep for words;* Romans 8:26. Regardless of the exact mechanism of action, I feel in my bones that everything Jesus did and does is with us, toward us, for us. That helps me live each day, and sleep at night. (That and falling asleep, holding a cross in my palm.)

So. Then, I un-garden and look for persistence. I am hoping to get the deck sealed/stained before the weather changes. (Which may or may not happen until spring.) In order for that to happen, some un-gardening needs to occur. To begin, the Black Eyed Susan vines and the Scarlet Runner Bean vines need to come off the 8-plus foot trellis on the deck. I can do that. I can stand upright and use my little hand pruners in every-single-hole in that trellis. Those vines worked to be there. Woven through by not just one, but half a dozen or more vines in every single hole. The branches, or little shoots off of the vine were not such a big deal. I could just pull them off when they were busy doing something else, but those vines? So, then I remember back to Jesus' *"I am the vine you are the branches."* (John 15:1-8).

I have a picture in my head of why Jesus used that image with his hearers: (1) they knew about that kind of tending....and the skills of the vine grower (God), and (2) they had seen how vines really truly grow. Just TRY to take down a vine! They are persistent in reaching, holding on, providing support for the branches,......and all that in one growing season in my yard. I have had now 52 growing seasons with the Vine Grower! With every single clip that I removed those vines from the trellis, I realized that I am being even more closely held and nourished by God. I clipped....and God said, "but I've still got you." I clipped....and God said "I've still got your daughters." I clipped....and God said, "I've still got your folks and your family and all those friends...." Wow. I've been out-persistenced. And, certainly, I have been out-loved.

A little good news....
Posted Oct 23, 2013 10:06 a.m.

The weather has made the yard look and feel like Christmas, and I "feel" like "Thanksgiving, but it is October -- and my news, for once, isn't scary! My heart CT scan came back a-ok! My heart blood vessels and perfusion is all normal! Hurray! I have a good heart after all! I am thankful for the nurse who called me with the good news, and who also, with care and caution, told me about the nodules and little masses throughout my lung fields. Dr. Puri and the nurse were not sure if I knew about them. Yes, I do, I said, and I am seeing a wonderful doctor in Iowa City about that. (She was relieved.)

A little reformation
Posted Oct 26, 2013 11:59 a.m.

This weekend Lutherans will celebrate the Reformation. Personally I feel a bit closer to that event (even though 496 years ago is a LONG TIME) because of my 2010 trip to Wittenberg to the re-built Castle Church and famous door, where the 95 Theses were nailed (posted) by Martin Luther. (This event is memorialized in a springerle cookie mold that hangs in my kitchen!) However, I think that reformation and renewal was meant to be a daily thing...and a living thing.
This is how I have and will be remembering and living the Reformation:
1) Springerle cookies have been made. Two flavors: Anise, and Pumpkin Spice. Two of my favorite molds have been used (among others): a bust of Martin Luther and a preacher in a 16th century pulpit. Pastor Greg Mayer loaned me a few new molds to try too, so that was a hoot!
2) Worship; four times in three days. Sunday at St. John's in Rock Island, and then daily on Sunday, Monday and Tuesday at Wartburg Seminary for their days of Reformation and Renewal (a.k.a. -- class reunion! Hurray!).
3) Emailing Dr. Mo with my questions about "someday" removing the fluid from my pleural effusions. Here's the thing....this week I have been

reading the Reformation Sunday texts....and keep coming up on John 8:36 *So if the Son makes you free, you will be free indeed.*

While I have never experienced "slavery," I think that there are little things each day that can "enslave" me. Probably this happens to most other folks as well. Certainly cancer could do this to me if I let it. While there is much that is beyond my control with the cancer, there are many things I can do to help the whole rest of my body be healthier......swim for exercise, drink water, worship, laugh, pray, create stuff, etc. It seems though that the current "enslaver" is worry. So, with the encouragement of scripture, I have told "Worry" to take a hike, and took a list of 14 questions about "what happens when a pleural effusion is tapped?" to Dr. Mo (via email), along with an update of other stuff, including that I have a GOOD heart. So there, Worry! Hah! You have been kicked to the street!

Hanging out with blessing
Posted Oct 30, 2013 11:25 a.m.

Yesterday I returned from Wartburg Seminary. Back from 48-hours with classmates....most of whom I had not seen since our three year reunion. This lil' trip celebrated ten years. This morning I woke up to rain on the way and that damp-cold-achiness that sets in the bones around that time. It was a good morning to catch up on some sleep, to read the past few days of newspapers and drink coffee until the pain medication started to kick in. What will I remember from those 48 hours?

~ Following wonderful Sunday worship in Rock Island, three beautiful worship services at the seminary -- honestly, being in the chapel there, when it is full of people who sing, takes my breath away....

~ Hope -- spoken in words of faith for and about Christ's church.

~ Sitting around round tables with my friends sharing and listening....all of those times together in the refectory or at a restaurant or wherever.....loving well and being well loved.

~ Hearing from Dr. Mo -- that he doesn't want to type responses to my 14-plus questions....he would rather talk to me...in person or on the phone, whatever I prefer.

~ Returning to my home....where my dear friend has cut and bagged ALL of my hostas and day lilies and last zinnias and gourd vines....and eight bags have been collected before the rain. I'm not sure how hard it will rain today, but I am already soaked in blessing.

Living every day
Posted Nov 5, 2013 10:58 a.m.

Today, November 5th is the 9th anniversary of Rod's death to colon cancer.
A lot can occur in nine years.
My 16 and almost-12-year-old are now 25 and almost 21-years-old.
Two high school graduations.
College searches.
Seven FAFSA forms (and counting).
One college graduation.
Birthdays.
Thousands of cookies baked.
Vehicles purchased.
A kitchen remodeled.
A pastoral call full of joys and sorrows.
Gardening.
A life-changing sabbatical.
Vacations.
Telling stories to one another.
A sarcoma diagnosis, surgery and chemotherapy.
Precious, loving, joyful time with family and friends.
Living. Living every day.

A birthday and "oh bother"
Posted Nov 11, 2013 10:34 p.m.

My heart takes a little leap. I remember that joy in the room 21 years ago when the doctor told Rodney and me – "It's a girl!" Sarah Elaine

Koppenhoefer celebrates #21 on November 12, 2013....tomorrow. She is a remarkable young woman and I celebrate her life!

However....while my heart soars, I am grounded. A little cold that started before Halloween has taken a lousy turn and I now have a sinus infection and bronchitis. I am toast. I now have an antibiotic and steroids, and an inhaler, and some codeine laced cough syrup. Oh bother.

Hopefully, I will experience "better living through chemistry" (as Rodney used to say) and I will be all better by the weekend, when we have a party for Sarah. In fact I am *planning* on feeling better. I just am....and I ask God to help me! Soaring and seated....and aching and coughing on the journey.

Thoughts on Thanksgiving...
Posted Nov 21, 2013 11:08 a.m.

This morning, I took my last of 20 antibiotic pills for my sinus infection and bronchitis. I do feel better. I am thankful for that. It feels pretty good to be back to just the "usual" aches. I've thought a lot about thanksgiving and what the most important thanksgiving is to me. I realized that I am needful of one thing, every week, should I need to stay home again like that. It is two things maybe, but they go together -- Word & Sacrament. That's it. Whatever else comes would be framed within the context of those words of God's love and forgiveness.....and the Great Thanksgiving: The Eucharist. That's what eucharist means.... Jesus took bread and GAVE THANKS. That meal is all about forgiveness and life.

Things that help, Part 12
Posted Dec 3, 2013 5:14 p.m.

Lately, after recovering from the bronchitis/sinus infection thing, I have been left with lousy feelings of nausea on and off through the day. I think that the prednisone played tricks on my body chemistry and has goofed up my metabolism. The nausea attacks when my blood sugar drops even a bit....and/or when I am riding in a car...and/or when I watch a 3-D movie on a very large screen. Oh bother. Unfortunately, my shortness of breath with simple things (a.k.a., tying my shoes, lying down in bed, bending over to empty the clothes dryer, or anything that makes my lung space go down or my heart rate go up) has worsened. With this, there is also some lung pain which comes and goes. Oh bother.

Oh bother is actually a code word for "occasional freak out" or "cry at the drop of a hat." The latest hat to drop was the movement of the calendar from November to December. Oh bother.

It seems that being "in the month" in which my next set of scans will occur is enough to distract me from productive or joyful pursuits. This has to turn around. This does not fit with my over all plan of enjoying life and living each day to the fullest.

So, the list:

1) Play the piano...not the slow-moving-heart-felt-stuff, but something that rings of mission and hope and has a good beat to it. My counselor reinforces that this regular music making has solid research behind it as well, as a way to "be well." (Be well...those are my words there, as I can't come up with another way to express the joy that has returned with regular music making.)

2) Return to the swimming pool. Taking about a month off because of illness was the pits. I have been back twice. I'm not fast, but I'm steady, and I hear God's voice in the waters of the pool... "Remember, you are baptized!" God has such a sense of humor, and a flair for exaggeration.

3) Be encouraged by the countless people who hold me in love and prayer.

4) Refocus with the words from I have said while I laid hands of blessing on the newly baptized and on dozens of young people who are affirming their baptism (e.g., confirmation). The prayer of blessing goes like this...."Sustain [insert YOUR name here] with the gift of your Holy Spirit: the spirit of wisdom and understanding, the spirit of counsel and might, the spirit of knowledge and the fear of the Lord, the spirit of joy in your presence, both now and forever. Amen."

I have been meditating on these words for two days now. Today I have been thinking about wisdom....and am more at peace about the wisdom I will need on December 17 to make decisions about my care and treatment. Today, my wisdom is to "not stew about it." Today my wisdom is to "not borrow trouble from tomorrow." Today my wisdom is to trust that the Spirit will provide me the wisdom I need, when I need it.

271

Scanning for Grace
Posted Dec 15, 2013 3:32 p.m.

Here is the "Reader's Digest Condensed Version" of this post:
1) I have my MRI and CT scans on Tuesday, December 17.
2) That scan day starts at 6:50 a.m. in Iowa City….and ends with a 3:00 p.m. visit with Dr. Mo.
 3) God has heaped up so much grace on me that it is a wonder I can even move about freely.
Here is the longer version:
Several weeks ago I took a call from a friend at St. John's Lutheran in Bloomington, in which I was asked to participate in a video project -- which they would use in ministry in 2014. In short, they were asking people to prepare and videotape a 3-minute "Faith Share" on one of the core values of the congregation. I was asked to speak on "receiving grace," and I said that I would be honored to do so. Last Wednesday, Paul Crownhart and Shaun Easton drove from Bloomington to our home to record the video. They were both very gracious and helped me feel quite comfortable as I spoke. After the recording, I told them something like this...
1) (I was crying….kind of relieved that I had managed to complete the taping without crying!)
2) That I was honored to be asked to do this…and that it was a blessing to me….especially because during this time before my scans it can be quite hard to concentrate on anything BUT the scans. And, focusing on how I have received God's grace in my life was (and is) an amazing thing to concentrate on.
3) That doing this project for St. John's in Bloomington gave me an opportunity to say my thanks to a faith community that has been instrumental in our lives as a family.
4) That it gave me the opportunity to reacquaint with a long time friend (Paul) and make a new friend (Shaun).
5) That they made the process VERY easy for me by traveling to my home.
6) I guess that the best part of all though was the opportunity to state, first to God, and then to others, what receiving the gift of God's grace means to

me. Although it reminded me a little bit of those "1-page" papers we wrote in seminary on incredible deep theological topics, there was none of the fear of grades. And not only did I get to decide what was key, and what would reach the widest age range of people, I had to practice saying it aloud. Pretty much the practice came because I had to get past the stage of weeping as I read it. Oh bother…

7) And….that truly, doing this sort of pondering is a faith practice I recommend to all; what a gift.

So what have I been doing besides thinking about "God's grace?" My shortness of breath, doing what I consider VERY simple things, has really increased. After talking it through with Eric, and carefully reviewing the previously established history I have with the tumors in my lungs, we think that the bigger issue for the shortness of breath is the fluid around my lungs (pleural effusions).

So, THAT means that I am truly ready to have Dr. Mo (or his medically/surgically skilled designee) *remove* that fluid and return me to a more comfortable way of life. I don't know if this will happen on Tuesday or if I will have to return to have it done. Am I freaked out about this? Hummm…..occasionally, yes. I do have an idea of how this is done, but being "on the other end of the needle" for this procedure is not my preferred location.

Regardless of what they find on those scans, I do know this, there are many more things to scan for in our lives that will never show up in an MRI or CT. Grace is one of those things. So is hope. So is faith. So are the prayers received. So is compassion. I have received all of those things in abundance.

Iowa City Schedule for December 17, 2013
Posted Dec 16, 2013 10:09 p.m.

Here is my schedule for Tuesday, December 17 in Iowa City:
6:50 Arrive in Iowa City and get right to the MRI area to prep for the scan
7:20 MRI scan
8:15 show up for CT, and drink their "purple Koolaid" in preparation for the CT

9:15 CT scan
11:00 Dr. Buckwalter
3:00 p.m. Dr. Mo

Oh bother....the results
Posted Dec 17, 2013 6:43 p.m.

So here is the scoop. A couple of tumors are about 30% larger. However the fluid in my left lung has increased greatly and has even pushed my heart to the right. (The usual position for the heart is to the left chest).
I will return on Thursday of this week for a pulmonologist to tap my left lung and drain 1-2 liters of fluid. I will return after Christmas to see if it needs to be repeated. Then... After the new year I will start chemo .....likely a clinical trial. We don't have information on that yet.

Home a little "lighter"
Posted Dec 19, 2013 2:04 p.m.

Home. That is such a wonderful word. Erica, Sarah, Mom and Dad traveled with me today to Iowa City....or rather, me with them, as they drove me and wheeled me.
The fluid removal procedure went very smoothly, and the doctors and techs were exceptional. A little over 1.5 liters (like about a quart and a half) of clear yellow fluid was removed from around my left lung. I asked "why yellow?" and the doctor said it is sort of like the inside of a blister....oh, I get it....sort of...The coughing that followed the procedure resulted in a bit of pain and nausea, but helped both lobes of my left lung do a lot of re-inflating. The upper one looks pretty good and the lower one is much better, yet not quite all the way open. In this one morning I've seen myself on the inside via CT scan results, an ultrasound, and a follow up X-ray. I still do have a heart, and now it is much closer to its original location AND my trachea has shifted back to midline as well -- that would explain why I couldn't breathe well before when I turned my head to back out of the driveway! I got a look at two pleural (lung lining) tumors that are resting between the ribs in my upper chest. I was told about pleural

274

tumors before but somehow had pictured "little balls that would be sucked right out with the fluid"....that is just not the case. These tumors are what are causing some of the chest wall pain, I guess. This realization was cause for a bit of a pre-fluid-removal-crying-episode. Sometimes that's just the way it is. It is what it is. So. Home. Breathing. Offering prayers of thanksgiving. I say "bring on Christmas."

Blue
Posted Dec 22, 2013 11:27 p.m.

Blue is not the way I hoped to travel these holidays, but that is what I have. I worshiped at a Blue Christmas Service this evening with two remarkable friends. I needed to be there. However, I am so very much wanting to be "other than blue." I want that for me, for my daughters, my parents, my extended family and many friends and for those around the world whose troubles I cannot begin to imagine. I know that I am not alone in this season....or in this blue-ness. So.... Let's pray....I think it is something like this....
Loving God, our coming newborn King,
We bring our only offering....the gift of our tears.
You weep as well...
Our tears are precious to you, even if they are signs of sorrow to us.
Receive them and us into your embrace.
Give us peace this night, and hope in each new day.
Amen.

The look of hope
Posted Dec 23, 2013 4:28 p.m.

Although the thermometer said One Degree this morning, the sun was shining brightly and has done so all day. How does that line go? "My future's so bright, I have to wear shades." That is a bit of what I feel right now, sitting in the sun in my dining room....The "causes" of the "blues" haven't really changed, but it seems I woke with hope.

275

Hope which looks like this:
Thankfulness
More thankfulness
Eating ever so slightly more than I did the day before
Reading the lessons for Christmas eve, while drinking my coffee this morning
Going swimming…and realizing it is a LOT easier to swim/water walk/etc. with two functioning lungs
Going out in the coooooollllldddd… and not having an asthmatic response
Preparing to make cookies with my daughters
Preparing to pray some time in the next day with a dear friend
Breathing without shortness of breath
Hearing from friends and family
Mailing some Christmas cards BEFORE Christmas
Excitement from looking forward to worship tomorrow night, and time with family in the coming days

The light shines…
Posted Dec 24, 2013 10:33 p.m.

The light shines in the darkness….and the darkness does not overcome it. John 1:5
This evening, after worship, and after take out Chinese food, my daughters and I shared gifts with one another. It had been a while since I had wrapped them (except for the ornament I finished knitting last night!) and I was glad that they were all in their places under the tree -- even without my "re-counting."
Now that the last cookies are iced and the plants are watered, and I am eating my healthy snack (apple), I'm thinking back on that present "counting."
Although the last week has been difficult on so very many levels, I still have my vision -- that is, I can still see by that Light that cannot be overcome by the darkness. What do I see? Or rather, who do I see? You. And you. And you over there too. Your prayers and encouragements and jokes and questions and sighs are gifts to ME -- and to all of you, too. For

this is true -- I am not the only one standing (or sitting, or lying down) in this Light.

This late afternoon, in a darkened sanctuary, we sang "Silent Night" by the light of hundreds of candles. It really only takes the One Light to light the room, but the company of so many is so beautiful, and so encouraging, and so warm on these cold days.

A look inside
Posted Dec 26, 2013 11:53 p.m.

Well, it is late on Thursday, December 26 that I write. From worship to travel to time with family and return to Rock Island this afternoon, it has been a lovely holiday. Although I was honestly quite afraid (after my "Blue Christmas Worship Service" crying fest) that I might burst into tears each time I saw another friend or family member. Rather, I smiled. I mean, really, how can I not smile to see such wonderful people.

So, Mom, Dad, Erica, Sarah and I head back to Iowa City early tomorrow (Friday, December 27) for a repeat x-ray and a visit with Dr. Mo...and truth be told, likely also a visit with Dr. Thomas or one of the other pulmonologists. They are checking to see if the 1.5 liters of fluid which were removed from my left lung have decided "good riddance" --- OR if some has returned. What I know is that I have had a week of such lovely breathing that I can consider it nothing other than a gift.

I have been getting lab results back almost daily for the last week through my University of Iowa online "MyChart" and I have learned a few lovely things....for instance:

1) the fluid had absolutely no cancer cells in it
2) the fluid was free of any infection

So, what will tomorrow bring? Hmmm....my guessing has me prepared for another fluid removal procedure....maybe even two (one for each lung).

The chemo plan...
Posted Dec 27, 2013 1:29 p.m.

We have been to Iowa City and are back. Mom and Dad are returning to Pontiac. The girls have both headed to nap. I'm eating leftovers, and watching the animals nibble on stuff in the snow in the back yard.

I didn't do any reading before I left this morning, so I took a look at the Gospel for this Sunday (Matthew 2:13-23)....where Joseph gets a message from an angel in a dream to get out of town with Mary and little Jesus....Herod was tricked by the wise-guys, and now he is out for blood....or baby boys, or both, with the plan of thwarting the leadership of this tiny new King. I never did trust Herod.

I can't say that Dr. Mo is an angel; however he and his P.A., Debra Ely, really are wise and excellent caregivers...and certainly want my healing and safety. My healing literally will involve "getting out of town" once a week, to go to Iowa City for chemotherapy.

These are the details as we know them:

1) Gemcitabine (Gemzar) will be the chemo. (It has been used in sarcoma, although it is more usually used in ovarian, breast, or pancreatic cancer.)

2) Most all of the eight or so possible chemotherapies for sarcoma of my type have about a 20% success rate for "progression-free disease"....meaning this is not likely to cure/remove my cancer, but has a 1:5 opportunity to STOP my cancer. (This is a very important area to consider in prayer....)

3) The chemo will be administered in my port (that I still have from over 2 years ago)

4) I will get the chemo at the University of Iowa's Holden Cancer Center infusion center....it is beautiful. We went to take a look today. (Last time I was an inpatient in the Clinical Research Unit of the hospital.)

5) The chemo itself will run about an hour and a half. Before the chemo, I will have an X-ray...and labs....and see Dr. Mo.

6) There was NO CHANGE in my lungs from eight days ago when the left side was drained. That is WONDERFUL!

7) Therefore, I did not have any more lung tap procedures done today. I can still have that done, even with chemo, if I need that in the future.

8) I will get to KEEP my hair after all!

9) This is not a clinical trial. I can be on this chemo for a year or more if it is working for me.

10) Dr. Mo has a long list of other chemos that we will switch to or try if this one is not doing the job.

Now I feel like I need a nap!

It will start...again
Posted Dec 31, 2013 10:05 a.m.

My chemo is scheduled to begin on Friday, January 3. (with lab work, X-ray and Dr. Mo visit in the morning, and chemo starting around 1:30 pm....following which I will come home.)

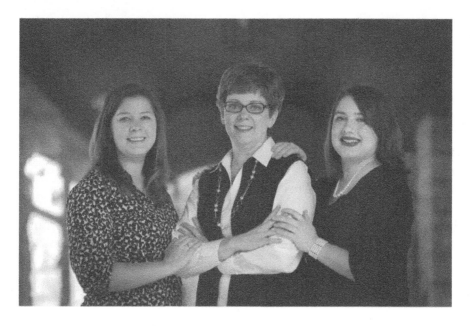

Pre-Thanksgiving 2013 – Sarah, Laura, and Erica

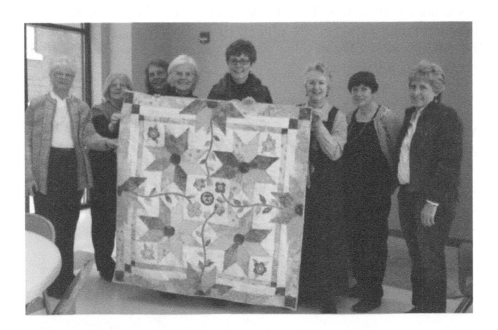

January, 2014 – "Son Shine in my Garden" quilt created by a quilting group of St. John's Lutheran friends.

L to R: Joann Dennis, Julie McCafferty, Karla Miley, Vicky Morrow, Laura, Dorothy Beck, Ruth Suman, Penny Logan.
(not pictured; Sarah Kivisto)

There are large sunflower images and small blue flowers made from bits of material from the baptismal quilts the group also makes.

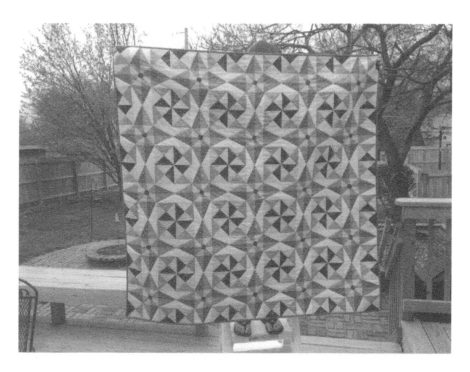

April, 2014 - The green five-foot-square quilt Laura made "with love" for Erica was a year-long-project. There are 40 triangles and one circle in each of the 25 larger squares. The pattern is Crystalline by Mari Martin for Connecting Threads.

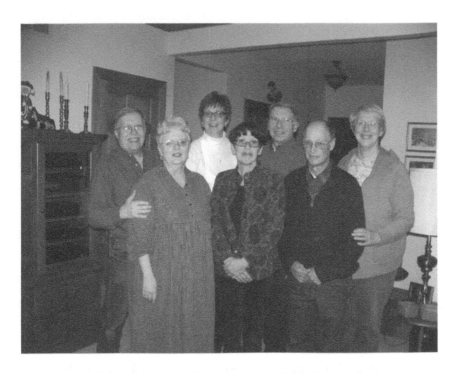

The Koppenhoefer siblings and in-laws.

L to R; Bruce Koppenhoefer, Diana Koppenhoefer, Laura,
Dee Brines, Steve Koppenhoefer, Rick Brines, Sue Koppenhoefer.

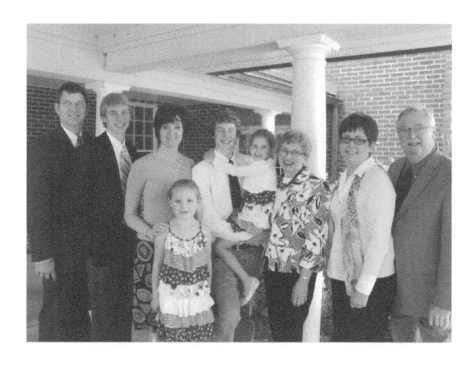

Mom, Dad and I travel to Mississippi for a visit with my brother, Eric and his family.

L to R; Eric Harding, William Harding, Katherine Harding, Amy Harding, Harrison Harding, Chelsey Harding, Marion Harding, Laura Koppenhoefer, and David Harding.

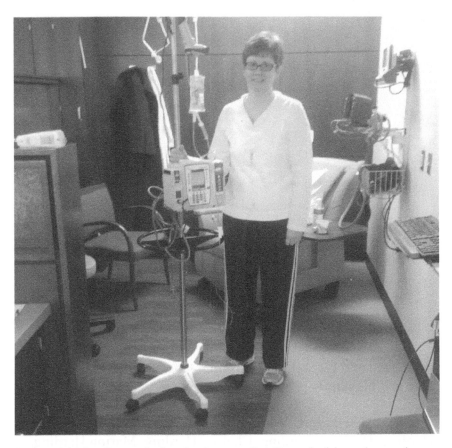

Spring 2014 – Laura is hooked up to the Gemcitabine chemotherapy, and ready for a short walk.

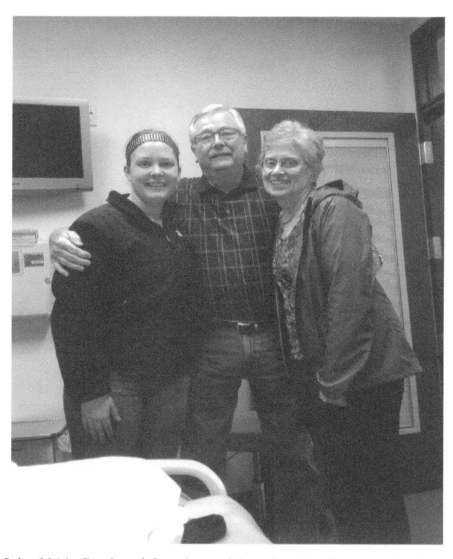

July, 2014   Sarah and Grandpa and Grandma Harding on a day at
the University of Iowa Hospital & Clinic in Iowa City, Iowa. The
day included lab work, a visit with Dr. Mo, and Gemcitabine chemo
in the Infusion Center.

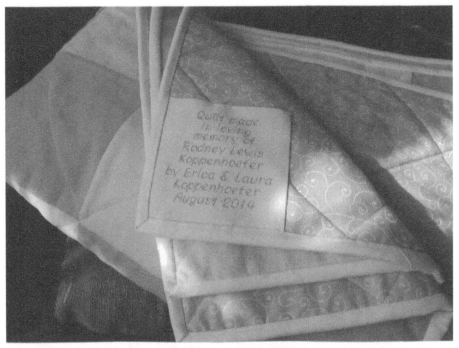

Erica's "Rod Quilt"

August, 2014 Laura and Erica pieced the squares for the top of the quilt made of Rod's yellow and orange golf shirts, and white dress shirts. The backing is a bright yellow print.

2014 UPDATES

Home...Thanks be to God
Posted Jan 3, 2014 8:36 p.m.

Picture the recliner. Me in it. Decaf green tea in a tall mug by my side. You know who this was a tough day for? The tumors. For me, for us, it was long. It was a lot of answers to a lot of unknown things. Probably tomorrow or the next day I will reflect on that more. For now, we are glad to be off I-80 (very windy on the way back), and back in our warm home. For now, I'll deal with the aching feeling that is beginning to kick in....not too severe, just present. I guess this is supposed to peak between 6-12 hours after chemo (which ran from 3:00 p.m. until 4:30 p.m.).

Update....after First Chemo (updated....)
Posted Jan 6, 2014 9:12 p.m.

I sit back in the recliner tonight...sipping on a tofu-strawberry-raspberry-crangrape smoothie, hoping it will ease my sore throat. Yesterday I had some brief witty thought of how to post the do's and don'ts of chemo as I was experiencing them, however, my witty streak either got sucked up by real-life, or frozen by this ridiculous weather. (...and I haven't even been outside other than to grab the newspaper.)
So, I think I will try a summary....maybe upon further review I will come out feeling better than worse.
1) I don't have a fever. (Updated: 9:30 p.m....I do have a bit of a temp...not high enough to call Dr. Mo, but high enough to watch)
2) I do have a cough...one that really hurts if the pain meds wear off.
3) I have a sore throat, but no mouth sores.
4) I wonder if I have a little cold.
5) The anti-nausea meds have worked well.
6) Almond milk is a no-go.
7) I have aches....which I usually have anyway.

8) I have checked in with Iowa City twice (following their post-chemo-stuff-to-call-your-doctor-about-list).

9) Dr. Mo is having me get an X-ray on Friday before chemo.

10) Erica's Corolla would not start after work today....and the tow truck came in about 1 1/2 hours instead of their 6 hour estimate. I think that man is a saint.

11) The girls made two trips to the pharmacy for meds for me, and have rubbed my legs and head and feet (not all at once), as have Mom, Dad, and Penny.....honestly, if I was going to find something to be addicted to, that would be it. That is healing touch....

12) Stacie and Penny brought communion to me and Erica yesterday. Best meal of all.

13) I have had two "declared" pity-parties. They were not surprising, but they are lonely, and the company is lousy....(I can't get away from myself....)

Things that help, Part 13
Posted Jan 8, 2014 10:01 a.m.

Time for another list. I know that it is early in the day (8:47 a.m.), but I declare that I am feeling better, for real. So, what has helped, you ask?

1) The story of Jesus' baptism. The words *"This is my son, the Beloved, in whom I am well pleased."* Honestly, in these days when I have felt so very lousy, the only thing that really helped was love....love that looked like massaging my head or feet....like helping me get food before the nausea kicked in.....like repeated trips to the grocery store....like filling the humidifier......like cleaning the kitchen....like checking in on me.

2) When I got my pre-chemo-education from the nurse and the pharmacist, they both said, "You may have diarrhea or constipation....but DON'T get constipation. But you may. But don't." So, today, as I was proving once again that I did not, in fact, have constipation, I was so excited that I just flushed the toilet when I was done! Yahoo! That is pretty funny, because I had also been instructed to close the lid, and to flush twice, to completely remove any chemo "waste" from the toilet. But no, not me. For that brief moment, I was just regular (pun intended) old me, going and flushing, without a care in the world.

3) I am, of late, a napper. I don't know if this is related to the cold or the chemo, but these have helped.

4) Being told by Dr. Mo that the fever I had was probably from a virus, and not concerning because I had not been on chemo long enough to have it drop my counts.....and, that I could take Tylenol for the fever.

Back to Iowa City

Posted Jan 9, 2014 10:39 p.m.

Oh bother.

I feel lousy again....even have a little temp.It was a gift for the three of us to see Trina and Dennis (seminary buddies who live in Claremont California at this time).... and then here I am again.I think it is a sinus infection.

Oh bother.

So. Tomorrow, Friday, January 10, Erica and Sarah are taking me to Iowa City....we leave around 9:00 a.m. with a typical schedule for the day.

Honestly I have no idea how this will play out. It might be a week off with antibiotics.....maybe I am even hoping for that.

Home.... No chemo

Posted Jan 10, 2014 4:36 p.m.

I think there could be several stories today, based on what perspective you viewed the day from. Here are a few:

Mine: I rode over to Iowa City with my daughters. I waited either very short or very long times for things. My blood drawing went exceptionally well. I started feeling lousy again. I started running a little temperature again (which I did through the night as well). I wore a mask to protect the other people. I talked through my week and how I was feeling with the Oncology Fellow (whom I had talked to during the week). She had not thought I needed an antibiotic but was changing her mind after she examined me and listened to my lungs. She told me that there was NO INCREASE in the fluid around my lungs -- YAHOO!!! Dr. Mo came in and said that my blood counts were still good enough that I could have chemo. I argued that I have a terrible sinus infection (which had gotten worse). He said it is because of his toxic drugs. I disagreed. He said I will feel better in a week…..and after he gives me another round of Gemzar, we will know if I felt better because of the antibiotic or because of the week off of chemo. I think I bet him on that (he seemed to want to shake hands on it…..although I did not put any money on the table.) I don't like the notion that I am betting against the smartest guy in the room…. I do like the idea of feeling better for a bit….OK, for a LONG bit. I will go back next week (on Friday) to do this all again, and actually have the chemo.

Sarah/Erica: (all of the above stands)….plus, parking deck 4 is huge….and has two areas that are identical to one another…..that are only accessible via a "tunnel" on one level….and the security guard's car is odiferous….and a car has not been stolen out of one of the University of Iowa's parking garages in at least the last 11 years…..and no, there are not security cameras to tell you who stole your car if it was stolen and not just parked in the secret double lot.

All the nurses: "That Laura Koppenhoefer has a remarkable weekly record of her meds, symptoms and temperatures….she must have been a nurse, and a super one at that." (This perspective is completely imagined…..I finally begged for acknowledgement of my skills with the last nurse of the day. However, I do have a completely great record. This record also compensates for what I call "chemo brain," which I may or may not have.)

Feeling good… And focus

Posted Jan 15, 2014 12:01 p.m.

I feel good today. I do. No fever. No cough. No sneeze. Aches mostly, covered by the pain meds. I feel good today. Now. I had sort of a feeling like I needed to get that written down right away, because it is true right now. This moment could be fleeting. Focus; the "in the moment-right now" kind of focus is what I seek. I read of John the Baptizer….busy about his ministry, but he knows that Jesus is out there and he prepares the way…Jesus is the focus. Single minded focus. I will say that this "healing" takes a lot of focus….and prayer.

Home again after Gemzar (#2)
Posted Jan 17, 2014 7:44 p.m.

It is such a wonderful blessing to have so many caring people, who work together to care for me. Today, the team included Sarah (my daughter) and Penny (my friend)….and great doctors, nurses, medical technicians, and a dietician. Before the chemo hits its peak starting sometime around 8 p.m. tonight, I think I will gather a few thoughts about what I learned today:

1) While I probably had a bit of a sinus infection kicker with that last chemo, both Dr. Mo and I are guessing that I am in that 30% of folks who have the "sinus pain -- cough -- sore throat -- and fever" as my chemo side effects. The throat "tickle" has started and I am keeping it at bay with hot tea continuously.

2) That the Tylenol I have been taking for extra aches and fever coverage is not helpful to my liver, which is having a bit of a struggle with the chemotherapy anyway. So…. I have been switched back to Ibuprofen instead of Tylenol. I've got a stronger med prescription as well, in case what I have doesn't cut it…

3) Dr. Mo is guessing that I will end up having chemotherapy for two weeks "on" and one week "off" to allow liver recovery time. That strikes me as lovely.

4) The dietician talked me through some soy options to use instead of milk.

5) My nurse, Chris, has really really funny cat stories.

6) Without exception, that nursing staff on the infusion unit is THE most kind in their care of one another that I have ever seen in a nursing unit. Every request for help is answered with helpful and gentle words.

7) Waking up, eating, getting out of the shower, getting dressed, getting in the Hilander, walking into the hospital -- all of those things seem to take an extra measure of courage in the morning when I am on my way to chemotherapy. I remember some of my favorite scripture. I am quite confident that my strength and my courage is not anywhere near enough to accomplish the tasks at hand. God's care and your prayers of support are so so helpful in just putting one foot in front of the other.

A little light....
Posted Jan 21, 2014 11:10 a.m.

Yesterday, when the snow had melted and then dried off the deck, I put a birdseed disk on the table....hoping it would be enjoyed by the birds before our squirrel buddies got to it. Shortly after I put it there, it started snowing. This morning I can't see it on the table at all. It is covered by two or more inches of new snow. However, a few birds have discovered it is there through their exploration of the under side of the table -- as they can see it through the open iron weaving of the table. Two birds have even flown up the six inches or so of free space under the table to peck at the bird seed disk and try to free up a few grains. I get that. Sometimes you have to work hard to find the good stuff, the good news, the morsels of hope.

Today is sunny; sunny, and especially bright with all this snow. It also happens to be a good morning for me. Granted I am using pain medications to help me come to this conclusion -- but hey, here it is – "I Feel Good!" No nausea meds needed. No extreme cough. No sore throat. No fever. No face pain. No extreme aching. It looks to me like the severe "yuck" that I had with the first chemo was mostly accentuated by the virus/infection. This is some good news. I've also had better experiences with eating in these last five days. Both daughters have helped by purchasing me some new products and trying new recipes. The whole thing makes the sunshine shine just a bit brighter today....and I am thankful.

I feel like those birds on the deck....I know there are grains there....hope there....promise there....and I want to find them and share them. So today I sit in the light....and pray for those who sit in darkness....that the Light would shine on them, too.

Yes, but no.
Posted Jan 24, 2014 5:03 p.m.

Yes....my liver is doing better.But no chemotherapy for me today, as my white blood cell count is too low.

Yes....I can leave earlier from Iowa City when I do not have chemotherapy. But I will not go very far, very fast, when I have already left the nurses and moved out to the reception desk to schedule my treatment for NEXT week and realize that I still have the access needle and tubing hooked up to my port (under my shirt). Oh bother! It takes a while to get back into the system even briefly, to get de-accessed.

Yes...chemotherapy will continue. But, it looks like chemo will be every-other-week instead of two-weeks-on and one-week-off. (This is Dr. Mo's thought as he sees what my blood counts reveal in these first weeks of treatment.)

Yes...I feel better today than I would have, had I had chemotherapy.But, I am pretty achy from this 'ol weather changing....snow is coming, people!

Yea, Chemo!
Posted Jan 31, 2014 5:11 p.m.

Home. Oh my, that word sounds so good! No weather issues leaving or traveling or returning today. Sarah made it safely home for the weekend. Now, praying Mom and Dad home safely to Pontiac is next on my list.

And -- the good news.

1) My labs were great!

2) The X-ray showed stability in the pulmonary nodules -- with perhaps a DECREASE in the size of one of them!!! Yahoo! (I cried. I hugged Mom and Dad. I prayed prayers of thanksgiving.)

3) The chemo went well...and was even on time, which is sort of an oxymoron when you are on the care-receiving end in a big, big system.

4) The lungs have a little bit more fluid on the left side than before, and the right side is stable. Let's get that fluid to decrease without having to have a fluid "tap"....got it?

5) I return in two weeks (Valentines Day) for my next chemo -- I told them that I "love" getting better, so that day is not an issue.AND...

6) I found out that I can go swimming if I feel up to it in these next two weeks! Hurray!!! (and by swimming, I mean water walking and such.) That will be good for mind and spirit.

All wrapped up

Posted Feb 1, 2014 10:00 a.m.

I am not yet 24 hours into Round #3 of Gemzar....I will make the 24-hour mark at 1:40 p.m. today (Saturday) and the 48-hour mark at the same hour on Sunday – Ground Hog Day, Souper Bowl Sunday (to collect money for the hungry in our communities), Super Bowl, Kitty Bowl, Puppy Bowl – or Sabbath.

There are a lot of ways to mark these days. I think I will mark them by what I have learned.

1) While I really appreciated making it through the process with maximum efficiency yesterday in Iowa City, I was also "gifted" with two extra hours of feeling really lousy while awake, instead of in a well medicated sleep. Oh Bother. However. I have learned that the way to address that is to ask for help, and surround myself with wonderful people. What did I ask for from the time I was riding back home, to sitting at home in my recliner? Warm blankets in the infusion center, and prayer shawls there and on the way home, and quilts at home. Comfort food all the way through. Leg rubs and foot rubs (especially because that weather front was hitting at about the same time). A grocery store run at 10 p.m. by Sarah for the saline nasal spray that can help prevent these nose bleeds. A borrowed DVD. Good stories. Caring nurses at the infusion center ....and caring family and friends at home.

2) I have less fear. In the months that proceeded my last quarterly scans, I had felt worse and worse. Pain. Shortness of breath. Aching. Decreased appetite. Weight loss. With all that came fear. Fear of a number of things, but among them, a fear of chemotherapy. My first experience with chemotherapy was quite difficult.Yesterday morning, it took a bit of a kick in the pants to move myself from sitting at the dining room table after breakfast to the "get ready, because everybody else is ready to take you to Iowa City." However, I went there without a fear of the chemotherapy. I know what to expect now. And, it also appears that the Gemzar may even be helping. Praise the Lord!

3) After last Sunday when I received the "Son Shine in My Garden" quilt (the latest in a gracious series of wonderful, prayer-filled warmers), I've spent some of every day covered by the quilt....and meditating on what it

says. It has written around the border, from *The Message* (paraphrase of scripture, which is one of my favorites) Joshua 1:9 -- *Strength! Courage! Don't be timid; don't get discouraged. God, your God, is with you every step you take.* I had taken a picture of the words *"Don't get discouraged!"* on the quilt another morning, as it was wrapped around my legs. Those words helped me think about my fear. (in the NRSV version, the words are *"Don't be afraid or dismayed"*.) For me, the dismay comes in my imagination on most days....sort of playing a "worst case scenario" game....and from isolation. When I get stuck in imagining what could happen, I get depressed. When I am depressed, I isolate myself and I am much less likely to ask for help. When I see those words again -- *"Don't get discouraged,"* I don't only hear "don't get discouraged in the big stuff," I hear it for the little stuff too....like "even though I feel crappy now, know that it will pass" and "you have so many loving people around who would help in a moment's notice -- ask for what you need! You will feel better -- AND encouraged!" Fear and discouragement are not "once and done" things. However, God's love is not a "once and done" thing either. There is new encouragement....there is renewal... each day, each moment, in community. If I need a warm reminder, I think I will just wrap back up in that quilt and read it again.

A little extra Iowa City trip
Posted Feb 7, 2014 9:45 a.m.

Last Friday, when Dr. Mo gave me the message to wait and come back in two weeks for my next chemo, I was thrilled! Two whole weeks away! Yahoo! However, I noted then that my left lung was giving more frustration with pain....shortness of breath on exertion....some related nerve irritation, and the like. Well, yesterday I said "Uncle"....or "enough!" and emailed Dr. Mo, relating my symptoms and requesting that the fluid be removed. (It has been about seven weeks since my first removal.) I just got a call from Deb, the PA (who is excellent), that the Pulmonary Clinic will take me for an appointment as soon as I can get there this morning. Super.

So, Erica is drying her hair. Penny is driving over from work. I am packing my "snack bag" (after writing this) and we will be off.

Home again and breathing easier
Posted Feb 7, 2014 2:39 p.m.

I am, exhausted,....and a bit sore; however, I am home. Mentally, I remember how to breathe using my whole lung space, however, some parts have yet to do their job re-inflating. In fact, that lower left lobe was so squished by fluid over time that I don't think it is jumping back into action very quickly. The 3-doctor-team removed 1500 cc's (that is a liter and a half, or about what they took off last time, less one cup.....and about four pounds worth of fluid or so). It will take a bit of time for the re-inflation process to do its thing. I was trying to think of something eloquent to say...and all I have is "Breathe." Just breathe. Anyone who has ever labored to breathe knows something of the preciousness of each breath. Anyone who has seen an infant take that first breath, or watched a loved one take a final breath has some appreciation of something we do every minute, every day. I have this picture in my head of the disciples, gathered up together, worried, mourning.....when Jesus shows up, and breathes on them. The one who wasn't breathing, was breathing again. The one who wasn't breathing, breathed the breath of the Holy Spirit on them. Truly God-inspired-life. I think that is the gift of each breath...inspiring God....

Bumps and blessings...
Posted Feb 12, 2014 2:10 p.m.

This morning I was feeling pretty good again. I had recovered from the last chemotherapy within about four days or so, but then I had about 2 1/2 days of recovery to do after the "lung tapping" (thoracentesis). The errands and activities of yesterday set so well with me that I decided to take my new (to me) vehicle and do quick trip for some Valentine shopping. As I returned to the vehicle after my second (and last) stop, I proceeded to open the door -- with my forehead catching the corner tip of the door. Other than what will likely be a bruise, and a drop or two of blood, I am fine. I sat there for a few minutes to take stock of how I was feeling, and how the "new door" obviously opens and closes in a different place in relation to my anatomy than all of our other vehicles. Lesson learned.

That got me thinking about the other lessons I have been learning lately -- especially related to quilting. I've made a number of things in the time since my diagnosis, but in the last few months I have really worked toward completing a quilt for Erica -- which is far beyond my previous quilting "skill set." It involves a lot of time measuring, cutting, pinning, sewing, ironing, and the like. I have also learned…

1) The value of having other people to talk to, commiserate with, and seek information from about quilting.

2) That sometimes the most beautiful things are not things I looked for, but rather found me. (This quilt kit was a gift from a sister-in-law who had it, but didn't want to make it.)

3) That liking what you do in the "making" makes the process more enjoyable….much more so than just liking the final outcome.

4) That it is rewarding to learn new things.

5) That I respond well to encouragement. (OK….some of this I knew already.)

6) That love is woven into every stitch of every project….not just what gets a bow on it when it is done and given away.

7) That there is beauty at every single step….and when I see the beauty of the individual parts, it is much more meaningful to see the beauty of the whole thing.

8) That making things of beauty for another person is also a gift to me, in and of itself.

9) That mistakes will be made along the way. It is a good idea to forgive myself and learn from them. The concept of "grace" applies!

10) That I can see improvement as I practice.

Last night I alternated between sewing blocks and watching the Olympics as I pressed seams open. I realized that what I learned applies to what I am learning along this journey with sarcoma……and with life. Perhaps quilting is one of my metaphors for life.

297

I recognize that I would never ever seek out sarcoma for myself -- or for anyone else, just like we wouldn't choose to clobber our foreheads with car doors. However, beautiful things happen in the middle of the mess and pain of life....and it is so so much more lovely to quilt/fight an illness/live, when one's eyes are trained to beauty, and one's heart is turned to God and others.

Things to love about a Chemo-Valentine's Day
Posted Feb 13, 2014 8:13 p.m.

There are so many things to love about a Chemo-Valentine's Day!
~ That the day was proceeded by three days of feeling really great!
~ That at 8 a.m. Erica and Lori (Harper) and I will leave and likely get to see eagles along the Mississippi!
~ That at 9:30 a.m. the people in the X-ray department will be able to look inside my chest and "see" that there is less fluid there than there was the last time I had chemotherapy!
~ That at 9:40 a.m. I will check in and have my lab work drawn -- and those nurses are just wonderful.
~ That at 10:40 a.m. I will get to talk to Dr. Mo and his wonderful staff....and he will use his best wisdom to direct my day -- likely to include the chemo that is planned. However, I know that he has my best health at heart.
~ That at 11:40 a.m. I will start chemo....and I tell you, those nurses make the difference -- really! Who would willingly go do something that would be guaranteed to make you feel lousier? I know that the goal is to feel better -- even be healed, however, on that day, in that time, those nurses become the face of encouragement and hope.
I have spent Valentine's Days in many ways...including some years of really sweet parties with my own little girls. However, I will not at all complain about a Valentine's Day spent at the University of Iowa, with so many people supporting me and committed to offering me their very best, so that I can be my very best.

It's sweet...

Posted Feb 14, 2014 7:21 p.m.

...to be back in my warm home...to have clear roads for the trip back from chemo (the trip there was messy with snow)...to have prayers and encouragement and people checking in with me through the day...to be approved to go ahead with chemo today, because my lab work was OK...to taste the chocolate covered strawberries from my sweet brothers-in-law...to have the boil order lifted from Rock Island...to receive the wonderful care of so many people at University of Iowa...to enjoy another Valentine's Day...to feel the love...

The truth about observation

Posted Feb 20, 2014 11:00 a.m.

Socrates is credited with saying "The unexamined life is not worth living." There is likely a lot of truth in that. There are blessings and challenges in that as well. So...this is what I observe:

1) That my yard is still covered in snow, even after two 40-plus-degree days, and it is currently thundering and raining on that snow.

2) That the feeding of the bunnies (and birds and squirrels) on my deck results in "bunny pellets" as the snow on the deck melts.

3) That Erica's advance work in the basement, of getting everything up on top of something "plastic" will pay off, because we already have water in the basement. Oh bother.

4) That I spend a measurable part of every day considering what parts of me hurt, why these parts hurt, medicating them to keep the hurting from overtaking my day, and communicating these three facts to the people who love me and are interested in my comfort every day.

5) That when I spend so much time on #4, I need to consciously spend time on other things to keep my life from being defined by pain and my response to it.

6) Philippians 4 has been an immeasurable help to me in focus and re-focus....

7) That although the pain I experience may be only measurable to me, the most effective relief of this pain is communal. If I spend my day solely

observing my left shoulder's response to rainy weather (because of arthritis) or to an over distended diaphragm (because of fluid build up around my lung), then I would miss the joy of receiving a beautiful Prayers and Squares quilt from my sister-in-law's parents' Methodist Church in Jackson, Mississippi.....or a Valentine from a sweet Sunday School student in Rockford, IL...or anointing and prayers for healing by a friend because I missed that day in worship, or monthly bouquet of flowers, or a hopeful stand of sunflowers coming out of my snow filled table on my deck...., or countless prayers in worship and confirmation classes, and at meal times and bedtimes.....and on and on. When I observe these things, I see a remarkable, beautifully woven web of care, and love, and healing. That web is a sign of community. That web shows the truth about God's response to my pain -- that healing happens in community. These are the things that are excellent and praiseworthy. And, when I see that web for me, it calls me to be a part of that web for others. To make a difference in someone else's life. To help be a part of that healing for them. This healing looks like love, poured out, over-flowing, splashing around, soaking in......observable.....true.

Transfiguration....I get it.
Posted Feb 27, 2014 11:17 a.m.

Some things aren't changing any too quickly here... It is still winter. Our lawn is still 95% covered by 1-12 inches of snow, and more is on the way.Tomorrow is my 5th Gemzar chemo in Iowa City, with my folks and Sarah joining me this time. We will leave around 8 a.m. and the pattern of x-ray, labs, Dr. Mo, and chemo scheduled as in previous weeks; with chemo probably starting some time between noon and 1 p.m. The chemo process itself lasts just a little over two hours. Then we will travel back to Rock Island and hope that more snow is a ways off. One thing is changing, though, that I know of -- the calendar. This Sunday is Transfiguration Sunday -- with next Wednesday being Ash Wednesday, and Lent to follow. Some preachers I know are puzzled by this Sunday with the image of the bright, shiny Jesus. I've always enjoyed it. I preached for the first time in my life on this Sunday at St. John's in Bloomington a year or two before I went to seminary.

The basic story (Matt. 17:1-9) is of Jesus taking Peter, James and John up on a mountain, where he is transfigured before them, revealing who he really is....with guest appearances by Moses and Elijah....and then when they are pretty much overcome by fear, telling them to get up and "don't be afraid" and back down the mountain they went to continue following Jesus.

At this point on my journey, I appreciate the words "don't be afraid" a lot. It doesn't take much for me to make an emotional trip to a place where I am more overcome by fear, than by "who Jesus is." I guess that is why this year my meditation is on (1) seeing Jesus for who he really is and (2) allowing myself to "get it" (understand that that vision is for me as well). I don't think I am alone when I say I love those times "when a plan comes together" or I "get it" -- it being some great understanding.

The "it" that I ponder right now though is "love." Two days ago was Rod's 56th birthday. He was 46 when he died. While there were many moments through the years of our marriage when we truly grasped the depth of our love for each other, during the time I was caring for him in those six months of his illness, we were blessed with many of those moments.

I remember times during the raising of our two daughters when I came to understand the depth of my parents' love for me and my brother, as we parented our own children.When I think of my years as an obstetric nurse, with each birth, I had that sure understanding of God's love for each child, each family, the whole world, as that first breath was taken -- or deeply missed.

I imagine God's longing for cancer researchers and doctors to have those "aha" moments when treatments and cures come together in the face of the brokenness of cancer.

I also imagine God's longing for us to know how much we are loved, regardless of what shows up on an X-ray, or on a grade slip, or on a W-2 at tax time.

I am spending a little more time writing about this today, because, with my sister-in-law and brother-in-law, Dee and Rick, I am missing their son, my nephew Joe, whose birthday is today. For some unknown reason, a few years ago, after Thanksgiving, Joe didn't "get it"....and ended his life. I know that Joe's action changes nothing about God's deep love for him.

301

Each year as I pastor I would tell people of God's great love -- at Christmas, and Easter....and every week before and after for folks who would listen. Today as I remember Joe, I tell myself, and you, and anyone who will listen that God loves you. Thinking that God nor anyone else can love you isn't the truth. Each of us are beloved people. Your life matters. You may not "get it" today, but that knowledge (and feeling) of loving and being loved can return. Ask for help. You are loved.

The end of chemo; day 5
Posted Feb 28, 2014 9:17 p.m.

I'm home from chemo #5 (Mom, Dad, and Sarah were my trusty sidekicks today)... I'm tired, but not feeling too lousy. I'm hoping that the "chemo-kick-in-time" and the "here-comes-a-weather-front-time" don't happen at the "same-time" tonight. Dr. Mo is still watching the fluid slowly increase around my left lung, and scheduled me to meet with a cardiothorasic surgeon to do an in-patient surgical procedure called a pleurodesis, where the fluid is completely removed via a chest tube and then talc (if I understand correctly) is inserted in that area to make the two linings "stick together" so that NO MORE FLUID can fill up around my left lung. I think this could be a welcomed improvement. The procedure itself is a ways off. Prayers and encouragements are appreciated!

Enough!
Posted Mar 6, 2014 11:59 a.m.

When is "enough," enough? That is the question that has been rolling around in my head for many many days now. I have probably as many answers as there are "situations" that the question might apply to. I ask myself this question as winter hangs on, as Lent begins, as my basement/drawers/shelves fill with "stuff," and as fluid re-accumulates around my left lung.
1) Enough! Enough with the fluid around the lung. Yesterday I emailed Dr. Mo and his team, who returned with a phone call within the hour and talked about how I am feeling....how even simple activities result in

302

labored breathing, how my appetite decreases with "less room" for food, and fluids. Even though it has only been four weeks since my last procedure (unlike the previous seven week stretch), it is time to give it a go again. So, at 10 a.m. on Friday, March 7 (tomorrow) I will get another temporary fix....anticipating that a week from today, when I meet with that cardiothoracic surgeon, I will learn much more and get the surgery on the books.

2) Enough! Enough snow. The two additional inches yesterday were unnecessary, in my humble opinion.

3) Enough! Enough stuff. I am completely confident that I have more than enough "stuff." One of my strategies for getting rid of stuff has been "just waiting." For if I wait long enough, "stuff" doesn't work or doesn't fit or doesn't have an emotional hold on me or I have already replaced it with newer stuff. All that said, that strategy doesn't get to an underlying unhealthy relationship with "stuff." I remind myself that my security does not come from my stuff. My security comes from who I am and more importantly whose I am.

4) Enough! Enough pain medication. My life has improved since I adjusted that amount "up" during my post-chemo days.

5) Enough! Enough food, shelter, insurance. There are so many people who are "food insecure" ....meaning they don't have enough to eat each day...or sufficient water or shelter or clothing or health coverage. This is a good enough time to be thankful (again) for this type of enough.

6) Enough! Enough stress. There are some days that despite having all I need, I am stressed out. Maybe I have picked up someone else's troubles as if they were my own to carry or "solve." Or, maybe I have forged ahead in my "worry" class. There is no reason to borrow trouble from tomorrow. Besides the "enough"s which I have already listed, I am completely confident that there is more than enough grace and love from God poured out for me (and for you, and you, and you) for each day. More, even, than the flakes of snow in my yard....more than the mountains of boxes in my basement, more than the fluid that crowds my lung and distends my diaphragm....all handy reminders that I am not alone....and there is enough of what is true and loving for me and for the world.

Better out than in...
Posted Mar 7, 2014 3:06 p.m.

This thoracentesis (lung tapping) procedure went quite well...and perhaps in honor of St. Patrick, the pulmonary fellow (educational distinction) was from Ireland, and the attending physician was pregnant with her fourth child and due in about seven weeks.

In short, 1300 cc (or a quart and a bit more than a cup) was drained from around the left lung. Better out than in.

Time again...
Posted Mar 12, 2014 11:40 p.m.

It is late...and really time for bed on Wednesday evening....I have done many things to get ready for tomorrow, but haven't shared with you all what is going on. And, I am realizing that it is every bit as important to me to have my lunch and meds and schedule and ride as it is to have your prayers and support through days of doctor appointments and chemotherapy.

Eric and Katherine (from Mississippi) are here to travel with me, Sarah, and Erica to a day that looks like this....

7:00 a.m. Leaving home

8:30 a.m. Appointment with the cardio-thoracic surgeon, to talk about the pleurodesis procedure...and hopefully to get that scheduled.

1:40 p.m. Lab work

2:40 a.m. Dr. Mo

3:15 p.m. Chemo #6 (the completion of 2 rounds.....in two weeks I should be having scans to see how it has worked.) (I sure hope this is on time....it is a very long day.)

Home
Posted Mar 13, 2014 11:24 p.m.

Home.....(since about 7:30 p.m.)At this point my "Check to See How This Chemo is Doing" scans are scheduled for about two weeks from now.The lung surgery to remove the fluid and "stick" together the two layers of the pleural outer linings of the left lung is scheduled for Tuesday, April 1.

A puzzle
Posted Mar 20, 2014 11:30 a.m.

On most days I like to read the scriptures for the weekend ahead. Today was no exception. It was the story of Jesus and the Samaritan woman at the well (John 4:5-42). In previous years I would have spent several days to a week "puzzling" over that text, wondering what it was telling me, and wondering what good news it had for all of God's people. Of late, I have taken up solving the puzzles in the morning paper....the NEA Crossword puzzle, the Soduko, and the Jumble. When I do them, I tell myself that I am keeping my brain active and sharp. Combating "chemo brain" or the regular effects of aging....or both.

Actually, I think that my actual every day life is full of puzzles, and I like the idea of solving a puzzle that has an actual answer. A puzzle that gets sewn up in a morning, or at least by the arrival of the answers in the next day's paper. My "actual" every day puzzle is a 7-day grid, which starts on Fridays (usual chemo days). On this grid, I record all of the medication I take and how I feel each day....achy, tired, nauseated, good. This week my puzzle grid has been more puzzling. Usually I can figure out the pattern for the week based on the previous week' s "yucky-ness." This week the grid is a wee bit shifted. I had chemo on Thursday rather than Friday last week. I've had some pain in the day time that I have usually had in the night. My intestinal system has been giving me some real grief (sparing details here). And, the shortness of breath that I have had in previous weeks is returning, just as it has before. My mind is constantly sorting out this puzzle of my body. "Is this symptom a sickness/illness?" "Is this symptom something that is a sign of worsening side effects as the

305

chemo builds up in my body?" "Is this symptom a sign that the chemo is doing its job?" "Will there be signs of improvement on Friday, March 28 when I have my scans but no chemo?" "Will this symptom interfere with my lung surgery on April 1?"

Most of the time, when I ask these questions I am "playing" a puzzle that has no answer -- at least no answer that day, or in the paper the following morning. When I play the puzzle this way, what I usually get is more stress. When I play the puzzle this way I spend more time being sad or worried -- and neither of those things help me "feel better" overall.

Fortunately, the Lenten devotion book that I am using in addition to the wonderful resource from Trinity Lutheran (my former congregation) has me pondering some wonderful comforting thoughts, and challenging questions every day. For instance:

~ How was yesterday? How is today? God is right next to you...share your feelings opening with God.

~ God speaks to us all the time....what is God saying today?

When I approach my "puzzle of a day" this way, I end up being more relaxed, being fully reminded of God's love and presence, and less pressured to answer questions that aren't mine to answer. I just saw in my mind's eye a GIANT Rubik's cube --- I never did like those much --- which has some of my sweat and tears on it, and I simply handed it to God, because God is right here, and said "It is your turn anyway." A weight is lifted as God takes the cube.

I still mourn the questions from time to time, but I am reminded that I don't have to puzzle them out on my own.

Time for scans...
Posted Mar 27, 2014 9:30 p.m.

Whether I pay attention to days as they pass-- or not -- scan time comes around again. Scan-anxiety seems to work its way in whether I want it to or not. Oh bother! In this past week, the opening phrase of my Lenten devotion has read something like "Well, God, I usually come to you asking for favors, but for now I am going to sit here and just be thankful for your love which surrounds me." Wow! That has been hard to do. I feel like I have a pretty long list of "favors" to ask. However, I have kept practicing. Today it was easier. As this week has taken shape, Erica has not been well, and I have less lung capacity. Sarah and I agreed that it is a bit of a three-ring-circus....and that we have several tents in the basement -- so, why not?! I just asked if I could run the cotton candy machine because I think it is pretty cool.

Stable....a beautiful word
Posted Mar 28, 2014 5:37 p.m.

All of the appointments today came and went, just as scheduled; except for one...Dr. Mo. We actually saw him about 30 minutes earlier....and his words were just as beautiful as his early arrival. His initial look at the CT revealed that the sarcoma tumors look overall "stable." What a beautiful word. Compared with the last scan in December, there was less fluid in my lung lining, however he estimates 5-6 liters of fluid is hanging around that needs out. So, everything is a "go" for surgery on Tuesday. Dr. Mo said that he wants to get a CT repeated a week after the surgery to see what is going on in the left lung. It could be that things are growing there that would cause a change in the type of chemotherapy. But for now, what we know is "stable." You know...sort of like you...holding me "stable" in Christ's sight along a rocky road.

Time to breathe...
Posted Mar 31, 2014 11:40 p.m.

Tomorrow, April 1, is time for lung surgery, but....

Today has included time to check in with my daughters....
Today has included time to get a chipped tooth fixed....
Today has included paying bills...
Today has included tasting steak from the grill and lemon cupcakes, made from scratch...
Today has included packing a suitcase and toothbrush....(and some camels and Action Figure Jesus with posable arms)....

307

Today has included telling stories and laughing with my folks and daughters.....
Today has included my Lenten devotions....
Today has included watering my plants...
Today has included complaining about how achy I am and wondering when it might rain.....
Today has included calls and texts and emails and prayers and acts of care by so many....
Today has included praying and crying with those prayers.....
Today has included a supreme amount of patience from those around me as they wanted to get ready for tomorrow, and I have delayed a lot of that work until the last moments of this day...staying in the moment of today.

A quick reminder....the surgery is called a pleurodesis....a chest tube will be inserted to drain out the many liters of fluid that have accumulated in the pleural space....a few other little holes will let a camera and instruments work in lining around my left lung. We pray that when it comes time to "re-inflate" that it does so completely, as that means they would be able to apply the medicine which would in effect "glue" the two layers of my lung lining together, and prevent further fluid build up.

groggy and grateful
Posted Apr 2, 2014 9:05 a.m.

The surgeon said it went well yesterday.The chest tube is still draining. I am still working on pain relief.

Home
Posted Apr 3, 2014 9:33 p.m.

It feels so very good to be home. The hospitalization held many challenges -- mostly related to severe pain. Today held more trials at getting up and going. I am on oxygen until my lungs heal a bit. I know that life will be easier without that chest tube!

Stuck together...
Posted Apr 7, 2014 11:10 p.m.

This can be good thing --- being "stuck together"...or not so much....

1) For instance, there is great hope that the surgery to "stick together" the lining of my lungs, which I had 6 1/2 days ago on my lungs, is successful in preventing further filling of that lining with fluid! They took out over two liters that day...wowza...

2) I also found out on an "up close and personal level," that my activity level is "stuck to" my oxygen consumption....I say this as I smile with a nasal cannula for just a 'lil bit of oxygen support in my nose.

3) Around that same time I experienced that my Dilaudid use for pain has a direct correlation with my ability to spell just about anything.....wowza....

4) And, I learned that just because surgeons CAN pass ALL of the drains, video cameras, and instruments through one little hole in my chest, most every thing on my left side is stuck to that one hole....so, big or small, it is still going to be sore!....wowza....

5) I learned that by getting up only ONCE last night for pain meds instead of TWICE or more as I had for the previous several days, I would have determined when I actually HAVE to get up tonight, in order to have enough pain medicine in my system for my travel/labs/CT experience tomorrow!

6) And (see #3) that is not only my ability to spell, but also to calculate medication intervals which is "stuck together" with Dilaudid use.

7) FORTUNATELY -- we are all "stuck together" in God's love.....family and friends, neighbors and caregivers, prayers and encouragers.....and because we are, I know that I come out in a lovely healing spot on the journey.

And we all said "Amen!"
Posted Apr 8, 2014 5:31 p.m.

Good news. All the tumors are stable. Both of the lungs are beautifully still inflated. I get one more week off chemo to continue to heal from this old surgery and then resume the same chemo next week!

A different Easter...
Posted Apr 16, 2014 10:46 p.m.

Honestly, I prefer Holy Week and Easter celebrated in a traditional way....Maundy Thursday, Good Friday, Easter Vigil, Easter worship...I love the whole thing. I love worship. I love leading the worship and I love worship in the pew. The thing is, I have chemotherapy tomorrow (Thursday, April 17). Public worship will have to wait until I have recovered from chemotherapy.

I am so very thankful that Easter is a "season"...there is a lot more Easter to celebrate.The other thing is, I need Easter. Not just this Sunday. I need it every day. I need it when I wake up in the morning and when I go to sleep at night. On "good days" and "bad days." All days. I need the word of redemption. I need to know there is nothing (life, death, height, depth, etc.) that will ever separate me (us) from God's love (Romans 8:38-39.) When I hear the angel's words to the women again *"He is not here. He is risen, just as he said."* (Mt. 28:6) I know He isn't there. I know that. He's with me...and you...and the world....until the end of the age. So, tomorrow, and the next day and the next are all little Easters.

It's time to get re-started on chemo. I feel a bit better each day....except if the weather is causing the "aches," but certainly I am recovering from the lung surgery. I know that my lung capacity is increasing. I am less short of breath. The inflammation around my lungs from the surgery is decreasing, and hence less pain, too.

Whew...
Posted Apr 17, 2014 9:36 p.m.

Home. Tired. Thankful.
The left lung is still inflated nicely....and the smile on Deb, the P.A., was positively beautiful when she heard nice clear breath sounds in areas of my left lung that have been way too quiet for too long.The stitch in my side came out with minimal grumbling. My blood work is right where it needs to be. My oxygen level was normal, even after a walk in the hall with the nurse -- so the oxygen supplies can be picked up by the supplier. And, every thing went smoothly with the chemo.

So what's up, anyway?
Posted Apr 26, 2014 11:03 a.m.

I think about the story of Thomas and Jesus and the disciples that many will hear tomorrow in worship (John 2:19-31). The disciples will get to see, hear and touch Jesus, but not Thomas. Thomas will want the same "proof" of Jesus' resurrection that they all got before he believes. It is a full week later when all the disciples (plus Thomas) are gathered back up in the house where they were when Jesus appeared before, and Thomas gets his "proof."
I'm left wondering if the disciples were living like "Easter people" or "Good Friday" people during that week. Truly, I think life is a mix of both. So, what's up anyway? Here's a short list....
1) I finished Erica's quilt. It is wonderful. I admit though that I am grieving finishing it. It is a bit like finishing reading a really great book where the characters have become a part of your daily life and you want the story to go on. I'm glad to have another project to go on to, but I will miss that one.
2) I've been sorting out which effects I am experiencing are a result of chemo versus a result of the lung surgery. As the days have been less rainy, I can feel that the chemo is easing up on me and I have more energy and am less likely to take multiple naps through the day. I'm a bit disappointed to have some nerve pain on my left side and abdomen from

311

nerve irritation during the surgery. I didn't have ANY when I saw the surgeon a week ago, so I didn't even ask about it again, but it has returned. The waistband of pants and the touch of shirts on this "normal looking skin" are painful. Hopefully this too shall pass. I have gone 36 hours without the additional narcotics that I have used since surgery, and that is a welcome amount of progress. (For a week or two I was up twice at night to take more pain meds.)

3) I am breathing. This is so wonderful. It is especially great to go outside many times a day for "crop surveys" and not have to worry about whether breathing during the walk is something I will have to worry about.

4) Sarah is finishing up her semester and preparing to move to a new apartment -- and preparing for two summer internships (and a few classes). I admit that technology is a huge plus for me -- texting and Skyping to be able to touch base with her and hear the excitement in her voice and see her as she goes through this time. However, she is also home almost every weekend. She works very hard to be with me for Thursday chemo treatments. It is great to have her home and have her support and care as well.

5) I'm sorting out what tastes good. I had lost quite a bit of weight around surgery time. Eating is easier now -- most foods taste better. My mouth has saliva again. The fluid around my lungs isn't there to keep my stomach squished all the time.

6) I think that listing these things out has helped me. It helps me see that I am making progress from the weeks I've had of post-Easter-still-locked-up-in-my-house (with pain). The world looks good out there. I want to rejoin it.

Let's do this...
Posted May 1, 2014 11:11 p.m.

I've baked some of my breakfast cookies to take. I've printed my med list. I've picked my clothing -- feeling strong -- black Adidas pants, white shirt, yellow jacket, yellow LiveStrong socks. Standard fare for me, sure. But not so much a uniform as a cross between "team wear" and "work out wear." In this last week I have thought more about the research needed to really figure out what to do about sarcoma. That is a team I am on. And, chemo, in most every sense, is a work out. Certainly I want it to "work" on me -- and it can be said that it gives me a "work out" on about every area that I have levels! There are a few other things that I will do tomorrow…as well as all the days when I'm not receiving chemotherapy. They are pretty straightforward, yet not simple. They certainly take a lot of focus.

1) Breathe.
2) Practice "presence." (Be here now.)
3) Ask for what I want and need.

Research team
Posted May 4, 2014 9:44 a.m.

This morning in worship, most Lutheran churches will hear the story of what happened on the road to Emmaus (Luke 24:13-35). It is a remarkable resurrection appearance story, and one of my favorite stories in all of scripture. At the outset of the story, two of Jesus' followers have left Jerusalem after the terrible events of the previous few days….Jesus' arrest, trial, crucifixion and burial. They have heard, as others had, the "idle tales" of the women who said they had seen Jesus (…they would learn soon enough that the women were right). And these men were talking-- discussing-- looking closely at everything that had happened that past week. Turning the facts around and around in their minds. Trying to make sense of what was going on. (The story goes on to have Jesus join them on the road next, and then become known to them in a shared meal.

Discussing what the disciples were doing is something that I miss from my time in "formal" ministry -- the reading, dissecting, prayerful examination, study of the Word -- especially doing it with others -- other lay people in study or with pastors in study, or in a classroom while in seminary, or in continuing education. I have always believed and experienced that God's Word is a living Word that is both timely to the era in which it occurred and was written, and timeless -- sharing hope and direction and life in an on-going way. To use more modern language -- perhaps we can be called a part of "God's research team."

313

That brings me to last Friday; Chemo day. I had mentioned dressing and feeling like I was part of a team. Black pants…white and yellow shirts….LiveStrong socks. (As I walked around the medical center I realized that I also had the colors of the University of Iowa Hawkeyes on!) I said that I wanted to be on a research team. It turns out that I am. While I was waiting to be called back to the infusion unit for chemo to start, Wendee, Dr. Mo's nurse, tracked me down to tell me that Dr. Mo wants to run a "cancer mutation profile" test on me. I said that when my primary tumor was removed that they tried to grow cells to look at the DNA but nothing grew. She said, "Well, that was 2011 and now it is 2014 and there is new technology." They want to look at the DNA to see if there are any gene targeted therapies that could work on my tumors. Of course, I said "YES!" right away.

I remembered Dr. Mo telling me several months ago that as my tumors were attacked/bathed in chemotherapy drugs they would change to find ways to try to grow again. That happened with the Trabectedin (first chemo). That could be happening with the Gemzar. (Similar genetic testing approaches have helped people who have the BRAC gene for breast cancer, for example, receive genetically targeted chemotherapy).

It takes about two weeks to run the many tests. So, I am hopeful that there will be more information on the next trip to Iowa City.

As I write this, I am about 40 hours "post chemo" and feeling pretty well. I have been more aggressive with my pain meds and have also had the blessing of some "good weather" days. So far, other than general "tiredness" my only painful times have been in the evenings for a few hours. I'm not in worship this morning, but I am studying the Word and offering thanks for researchers….for those men on the road to Emmaus who sorted out what happened to Jesus….for Dr. Mo, Wendee, and the countless others who are finding new ways to identify and treat cancer…. and the rest of us curious ones, who hope to see the face of Christ in healing of every kind.

Getting ready first
Posted May 15, 2014 10:51 a.m.

I'm taking a different approach to my "last day before chemo." I'm getting all of that stuff I need to do in preparation for chemo done earlier in the day. (I hesitate to say "early" as some folks I hold very dear have been up and working for hours by this time!)

For example, I am...

-writing this update

-choosing my clothing and setting it out

-making sure I know my schedule

-getting my medications ready (including seeing what I might need new or refilled prescriptions of)

-preparing my "Easy Does It" bag of stuff to do

-preparing my food/snack bag with everything but the refrigerated stuff

-getting one of my prayer shawls ready to travel with me (even if it is 90 degrees out, I still get the chills at some point from the chemo)

My usual preparation has included all of these things, but I have pushed it to the last hour or so of the night before -- sort of like I am trying to squeeze all of the lovely "let's not think about chemo and cancer type of living" out of the day/week, and then prepare.

But this morning as I read the Gospel text for this coming Sunday, I heard the familiar words from John 14:1-14 *"Don't let your hearts be troubled.....I go to prepare a place for you...."* Granted, as a pastor, most of the time I read this Gospel was at a funeral. I think I like the term "celebration of life" better. In fact I think it fits here. When all of the tough stuff is already handled -- the hard work is done -- we can just focus on living. Jesus offers comfort (amongst many things) to his disciples when he talks to them here. Sort of saying, "You really have nothing to worry about in this life or the next because the Way is ready. I'm handling the really tough stuff ahead of time, and the Father has the house all ready for folks to just show up -- you don't even have to bring a dish to pass...the feast is ready."

So, I guess that today I want to live like the prep-work is done, and see what the rest of the day is like. I think it will be beautiful.

315

3 things...
Posted May 16, 2014 6:00 p.m.

1) It worked out beautifully to get all of my "stuff" ready to go early on Thursday. I would liken it to writing a sermon early in the week, so the rest of the week is left to enjoy. So, I will do that again.

2) Mom, Dad, and I got home a little before 4 p.m. This is especially amazing as when I checked in at the Holden Cancer Center they didn't have my name in the computer for labs/Dr. Mo/chemo AT ALL today! Go figure! Fortunately, I had a copy of the order and the schedule card from two weeks ago -- and they got me scheduled in very quickly for everything -- AND gave me a $5 gift card to the coffee shop for the trouble. I learned that the cancer mutation profile is not completed yet....and learned that likely there is not a chemo that is developed to match what I have -- HOWEVER, things are changing within the "years" as opposed to "decades" in cancer treatment. Chemo went fine and I am just the "usual-post-chemo-tired-and-achy," so all is well.

3) Dad and Mom tracked down two Gourmet Rice Krispie Treats for me in the cafeteria. All is right with the world.

"Now you see him...."
Posted May 29, 2014 11:05 p.m.

Today is Ascension Day.....the "Now you see Jesus....Now you don't!" (....because he ascended into heaven!...) However, I find that the last two weeks have left me with many more opportunities to "see" Jesus, than not. The biggest adventure of these weeks was to travel with my parents to New Albany, Mississippi for my nephew Harrison's high school graduation. Prior to that trip (about 530 miles or so from Pontiac, IL where my folks live), my longest trip had been to the Bloomington-Normal area for my nephew Rob's wedding two weeks before. Other than traveling to Iowa City at least every other week, I hadn't been even that far away since Christmas! I'll just say that being able to breathe more easily since my April 1 surgery is a HUGE plus! Whether I am at home or away, I am continually surrounded by people who love me and do everything they can to make my day to day life easier. And you know what? It works!

Pathway, prayer, and pledge
Posted May 30, 2014 7:05 p.m.

It is about 5:30 p.m. I'm home from chemotherapy. Mom and Dad have headed home to Pontiac. Erica has fed me a tasty supper. Sarah is driving here from Bloomington-Normal after a long week. As my folks left, we laughed a bit about how I might even "begin" to condense what Dr. Mo had to say today in the half hour or so that he spent with us....informing, caring, encouraging, explaining, teaching, requesting and imagining.... Wow. What a mind.

1) Pathway. The Cancer Mutation Profile is completed on me. Done by Dr. Aaron Bossler, MD, PhD of University of Iowa. (A test on 50 genes that show up in the cancers Dr. Mo works with, that was developed by the two of them....with a $10,000 grant....and now costs only $50 a test. What a true bargain.) It appears that the mutation I have (a switcheroo of two proteins in the DNA) has disrupted the "Wnt/beta-cantenin pathway." Right now, this pathway is being studied and corrected in trials on mice with synovial sarcoma. It could be to human trials in about a year. This "pathway" mess-up is also found in some liver, pancreatic and endometrial cancers and central nervous system tumors. Dr. Mo says it looks like I am the first one to have it show up in sclerosing epitheloid fibrosarcoma. (However, there aren't many of us....and I don't think many people have looked.)

2) Prayer. I had told Dr. Mo that I've asked many people to pray for researchers. He specifically asked me to keep that up...and to pray for the whole thing.....including and especially for funding for research. (He talked a bit about his frustration that people who play with balls and get them from one place to another (name your sport) make millions of dollars....and he said that with 1 million dollars "He could just soar....." I believe it. That brings me to #3.

3) <u>Pledge</u>. We talked together about fundraising. Dr. Mo said ANY donation is needed...$1. $3. $20. $1 million. All of them. People can donate right to University of Iowa and direct it to sarcoma research...and specifically to Dr. Mo's research and he will put it to use. $1 tests one gene for a patient like me. $10,000 funds another research study.
He said "You could raise money and send it in, or people can go online and donate.) I pledged to him that I would pray about that.

"Babies and the river"
Posted Jun 3, 2014 9:02 a.m.

I am now headed toward 4-days (96 hours) post-chemo. After that first evening following chemo, I had a really lovely Saturday. Then the "bus parked on me....and the wheels fell off...so, it was stuck there." Yuck. However, last night I slept and my low grade fever passed, so I think I will gradually be on the mend now.

 Through this time, a simple story that Dr. Mo told me and my folks has been replaying in my brain:
One day two doctors went out for a walk along a beautiful river. They enjoyed the peace of the place and the beauty surrounding them. The river was beautiful as well. One of the doctors started looking closely at the river and noticed something floating in it....then more things floating in it! What was it? They were babies! Really! Worried for them and their safety, the doctor ran to the river's edge and started pulling babies out of the river and making sure they were placed safely on land, and breathing well. The other doctor just watched as the first doctor pulled out baby after baby. Then that second doctor continued his walk upstream along the river. The first doctor couldn't believe it! Why wouldn't his friend help him save those babies? He needed help, after all. The second doctor said -- you keep pulling those babies out of the water! They need you! For me, I'm going to go upstream from here and figure out why these babies are getting in the water in the first place and put a stop to that. Then you won't have to worry about babies in the water ever again!
Dr. Mo said, "That is the difference between me, your oncologist, and my colleagues, the researchers. I pull babies out of the water and treat them.

318

The researchers are committed to making sure babies never get put in the water again. Until that is figured out, we are both needed." Whether we are two weeks, or 52 years old....we are all somebody's baby.

Off the top of my head...
Posted Jun 7, 2014 11:15 p.m.

This weekend the church in some ways celebrates its birthday....with the arrival of the fire and wind and presence of the Holy Spirit on the disciples. Their experience was the ultimate "Rosetta Stone" of the church, when they started speaking in the many languages of the many many people who had made pilgrimage to Jerusalem. They were about to take the Good News on the road. The language skills and the gifts of the Spirit were essential.

I've written a lot lately about Dr. Mo and his staff....as well as those who are leaders in research in medicine and related sciences. (I'm still praying about how I might help to raise funds.) I am still overwhelmed by the "language" of science that was used in the cancer mutation profile which I read for the first time last week. Lately, though, I am finding I need a little help with another sort of language....I am guessing that it is the sort of language spoken by others who have experienced cancer treatment. There is a bit of me that is embarrassed even to mention that I could use a little support with this....there are so many bigger fish to fry than this one, but, oh well.

I am losing my hair. It is by no means "gone," but it is very much thinning.We didn't talk about hair loss at the beginning on this treatment because it really was not expected. And for the first three months of treatment, I didn't have hair loss. Then I had a month off for lung surgery and now have had four more chemotherapy treatments.....and, well, the "slim chance" of losing some hair seems to be occurring. I've had a feeling like a day-old-sunburn on my scalp for about a month. (No, I don't have a sunburn...) For a week or so I've really wondered if my hair was thinning, and have spent an inordinate amount of time with two mirrors and a comb to count my hairs for myself. My hairdresser confirmed the hair loss....although I don't think most folks would think anything was different to look at me.

Outside…and inside too…there are changes. Hopefully, on Thursday the 12th, when I have my next scans, we will learn that this chemo is effective at reducing more than just my hairs on my head! So, I've told a few people about this….and now I tell you….and try my "comb over" skills and my blow dryer on a lower setting. I'm ready to check in with my Facebook sarcoma group colleagues for tips. Maybe on Thursday I'll get an idea if I need to plan for a wig or just styling tips. (I could really use tips on how to deal with the scalp pain…especially as the area affects the top of my head, down to about an inch from the top of my ears….sort of a bad "bowl cut" area).

Again….there are so many folks going through so much tougher things right now…and this is hair….but I think God had those counted, and that there are people no further away than my computer keyboard who can speak a language of good news for me.

It's about time
Posted Jun 11, 2014 7:15 p.m.

It's about time….

1) that I could sit outside on a clear blue evening and type this up….in my deck swing….while overlooking the recently stained and sealed deck and fence….while appreciating the flower pots of yellow, purple, white and green growing beauty.

2) that I ponder time itself. I'm reading "Mrs. Lincoln's Dressmaker," and I am struck by the events of the time of the Civil War….and that it started 100 years before my birth -- 1861. And, now I have lived over 50 years (52 1/2 actually). One of my spiritual and mental health practices since my diagnosis is to "be present" in the time that I am in. It also helps me enjoy the beauty that surrounds me right now. And that increases my gratitude, moment by moment. I am much less likely to take things like a simple trip to Kohl's (where I was the driver), or wrapping carefully chosen presents, or a game of cards, or a table full of friends for granted, when I am in the moment. However, looking back, way back, brings gratitude as well. As I read of thousands dying of typhoid fever and infection and many more thousands dying in war, I give thanks for advances in civil rights…and medicine….and public works….and pray for peace.

320

3) that I don't know the number of my days….but I hope to continue to make the days ahead for people with sarcoma just a bit better.

When you get what you hope for…
Posted Jun 12, 2014 5:12 p.m.

The morning had an early early start. Fortunately Dad seemed wide awake for the drive. The rest of us were pretty sleepy. We progressed through the morning seamlessly….the waiting rooms and staff and tests all familiar. Then we sat in another waiting room and waited for Dr. Mo. Instead, Dr. Michael (a doctoral fellow originally from Russia) came in to go through my physical concerns and questions….and talk about my CT scan. He pondered that my scalp pain is neuropathy and ordered some medication for that…and a "head CT" in two weeks. I have some odd sensations around my heart when I climb steps and the like…..and a "echocardiogram" is ordered for two weeks from now, too. I talked about the pain in my left rib cage and he went on to talk about my scans….and his interpretation that the primary tumor in my left lung is growing slightly. It wasn't what we wanted to hear, but I was in no way surprised. I guess that this is what I had prepared myself for. He mentioned some clinical trials and went to get Dr. Mo.
Then, Dr. Mo came in, leading Dr. Michael and said "Nope." He disagrees. Dr. Mo thinks that primary tumor is stable, and because it is not hard like a softball, for example, that it is free to change shape with my breathing and position changes. And, that it is actually not growing….and some of the tiny tumors on the other lung field are perhaps even a bit smaller. Really! He said that. Stable, and a bit smaller. Well, THAT made me cry. That wasn't what I was prepared for…..that was what I hoped for. The chemo stays the same. The hair will likely just be a bit "thinner in number" but not fall out completely.
Breathe.
I guess it gives me pause to consider the difference between what I prepare for….and what I hope for. I am finding that it takes every bit as much courage to hope for a better outcome as it does to prepare for a difficult outcome. So, in two weeks, when I come back for yet another chemo (having recovered from the one I got today), they will look deep

321

inside me again....this time for a heart and a brain. I think it is my Wizard of Oz day. I will try to bring my courage....which isn't so hard to do. For, I find that my courage comes with the presence of Christ.

Sources of joy...
Posted Jun 13, 2014 9:30 a.m.

Yesterday a dear friend wrote to me and mentioned Psalm 16. It was a part of her study with a group of people and it was how she thought of me and my writing. Today I've studied and prayed Psalm 16....what a joy! Today also begins the Northern Illinois Synod Assembly at Augustana College (two blocks from my house). Last year I attended for a bit. This year, because of the timing of my chemotherapy, I won't be able to attend.

However, I have had years and years of amazing experiences at assembly....enough to last for a lifetime, for sure.

I pray for those attending assembly this year....for our Bishop Gary Wollersheim, for the synod council and committee leaders, for the worship and music leaders, for the prayer leader, for the Bible study leader, for those from St. John's Lutheran in Rock Island who are providing hospitality, for those running audio/visual and taking photos.....and especially for those who are attending for the first time. May your life and faith be enriched by this worship and serving.....and may you be overwhelmed by the kindness of others in this expression of the church. I look forward, with joy to your stories!

I also look outside and see the newly planted garden....planted by Erica, who graciously accepted my "back seat driving-- oops, I mean gardening" as she turned soil and planted seeds and herbs last evening. Except for the gnats, and the limited energy from "10-hour old" Gemzar coursing though my veins, it was a most joyful way to spend a bit of my evening.

Today, I also rejoice in having had Erica, Sarah, Dad and Mom with me yesterday "in person," and countless people in spirit -- all evidence of "Jesus with skin on" (Christ's loving spirit) for me. I am so very blessed. And while seeing a "good sized tumor" in my left lung doesn't bring joy, seeing ample space for AIR brings great joy...now at 2 1/2 months after my lung surgery and it is still working! Oh my how I appreciate breath.

From Psalm 16;
6 The boundary lines have fallen for me in pleasant places; surely I have a delightful inheritance.
7 I will praise the LORD, who counsels me; even at night my heart instructs me.
8 I have set the LORD always before me. Because he is at my right hand, I will not be shaken.
9 Therefore my heart is glad and my tongue rejoices; my body also will rest secure.

Having a purpose...
Posted Jun 17, 2014 11:06 a.m.

Yesterday was a regular day.
One daughter away at college.
Another daughter away at work.
One hour spent on a stool in the landscaping pulling weeds.
Another spent hand sewing the binding on quilted placemats.
One hour spent cleaning the kitchen.
Another spent knitting a washcloth with leftover yarn.
A crossword puzzle finished.
The mail sorted.
A book read.
Medicated so that I don't hurt anywhere....but I also can't drive anywhere.
I can admit that I am bored on a regular day. Boredom is a luxury.
It means that I don't hurt too much. It means that I can breathe.
It means that there are things I can do, like sort receipts, or scan pictures into the computer, or sort through things in the basement (if I wear a mask), or clean the refrigerator or the junk drawer. But of course I'm not doing them....Maybe I am just "saying" I am bored, because that way I can hide from how much I am wrestling with my purpose. There is something there in addition to my roles as mother, daughter, sister, sister-in-law, aunt, friend.
What is it that I can do to make a difference for people who have sarcoma?

The Wizard of Oz...and Iowa City
Posted Jun 25, 2014 11:31 a.m.

This morning finds me in the dining room....feet up....coffee consumed.....and watching the birds feast at the bird feeders and drink from the bird bath. They offer quite a show. They also remind me.....of Matthew 6.*25 "Therefore I tell you, do not worry about your life, what you will eat or drink; or about your body, what you will wear. Is not life more than food, and the body more than clothes?*
26 Look at the birds of the air; they do not sow or reap or store away in barns, and yet your heavenly Father feeds them. Are you not much more valuable than they?
27 Can any one of you by worrying add a single hour to your life?
Yep. Don't worry. Really. It doesn't add anything.
Tomorrow is my Wizard of Oz trip to Iowa City.
I say so because "they" will be CT scanning my head to see if I have a brain (Scarecrow) and performing an echocardiogram on my heart to see if I have a heart (Tin Woodsman). I know that I already have courage (Cowardly Lion). I've been practicing courage for years now.
 Actually, the reason they are performing the tests is that:
1) They have never scanned my head....and I have that neuropathy (nerve pain) on my scalp.
2) I have pain near my heart because that is where one of the tumors in my lung hangs out. And it has been over six months since we got a "you have a great heart" exam.
So, these two things will be added to the otherwise busy and *long* day.

The time between Thursdays
Posted Jun 25, 2014 1:59 p.m.

I can't say that Thursdays are not important, but there is so much more to life than what happens in Iowa City. In fact....often, I am reminded that the stuff that happens in between happens on holy ground.
So, here are some of the places where I've found that holy ground.....

~ around the island in the kitchen, making home-made pizzas with Sarah and Erica,

~ at the dining room table, with a bunch of my girl friends, and with my daughters, and with my folks,

~ at Comedy Sports, with my girl friends or a bunch of my family,

~ outside in the shade, in weekly prayer with my friend Penny,

~ at Dot's Pots with Sarah and her friend, looking for things to add to our succulent gardens,

~ at the dining room table, taking turns working on the daily crossword puzzle with Erica,

~ on the computer via Skype or on the phone, visiting with friends and family who live at a distance,

~ at Schwiebert Park sitting in the shade of a pavilion or walking through the splash pool after dark,

~ plotting a birthday surprise with Mary and Penny for our friend Stacie, which resulted in some of the cutest penguins I have ever seen,

~ sewing or "fixin" to sew with Penny and then with Erica,

~ on the phone with a daily check-in with my Mom,

~ crop surveys of the yard,

~ African Violet reports via picture text message from Sarah (she is an African Violet "whisperer"),

~ worship on Sundays with Penny and Nancy, Susan, and Rev. Stacie Fidlar….and all the good people of St. John's Lutheran in Rock Island.

A brain at least!
Posted Jun 26, 2014 7:57 p.m.

I am still hooked up to chemo in Iowa City. It has been a long day. It is now almost 12 hours since we arrived. Whew!
In short, I have a head with a healthy brain. Whew!
And I have heart but no results on the test of it.
And now...I am done.

Well watered....
Posted Jun 30, 2014 11:46 p.m.

Tonight, I write to the sounds of over an inch of rain "already" at my folks' house outside Pontiac, Illinois. This is good. The corn and the beans need the rain. My elder daughter reports that our home in Rock Island has received three inches of rain (in two storms) this afternoon/evening, to add to the 1.5 inches yesterday! Perhaps if I was willing to wait a bit longer, I could have used the flood waters of the Mississippi to travel to see my brother and his family in Mississippi this week. However, we (my parents and I) are in a bit more of a rush, as we would like to spend some vacation time at Eric and Katherine's lake house this week. Ahhhh.....water. The thought of floating on the lake in the sunshine makes me smile already.While I think that the notion of baptism as "once and done" is exactly right theologically, I believe that Martin Luther's notion of renewing one's baptism every day is also exactly right.... So, as I float the rest of the week away, let's all give thanks for God's love that never dries out.

More and less...
Posted Jul 9, 2014 10:02 p.m.

Well....last week on the lake in Mississippi was wonderful! I spent time floating on that beautiful water every day. And, I played MORE Disney Princess Uno and Mexican Train Dominos, and laughed MORE each day....it was a hoot.

One un-welcomed MORE has been swelling in my feet and ankles and shins -- especially on my right side. Even with compression hosiery and watching my salt intake and elevating my feet any time I could, it didn't seem to improve. So, I decided to take LESS ibuprofen (e.g., Advil, Motrin)....as in none of it. (I had been taking it around the clock for several months to help with chronic pain. A few years ago I had noticed a correlation between that medicine and fluid retention. Within a day I was improving, and now I don't just have LESS swelling, I have none...even after a day that included walking and standing! I am really looking forward to sharing this news with Dr. Mo.

Today at my hair cut appointment, my hairdresser told me that although I still have thinning, I now have MORE hair! Tiny hairs are growing in! Ta-Da! I didn't even know I had it in me.

Our home will soon have MORE people in it as my folks and Sarah are on the way here , and are going to my appointments with me tomorrow in Iowa City. Fortunately, we will get MORE sleep than our last visit, as we get started later in the morning.

The ups and downs of updates
Posted Jul 10, 2014 10:04 p.m.

1) Major update: My heart is just fine. Yahoo!

2) Mom, Dad, and Sarah did a very fine job of hanging with me through the day. Everything went smoothly and we got finished in record time....

3) Everybody at U of I was impressed with my skinny ankles. Of course I did tell absolutely everybody, and they probably take some sort of oath about expressing joy with patients who are joyful.

4) The truck (a.k.a., bus) has arrived and parked on me (...this means I feel yucky).

Next time, would someone please remind me to put up "no parking" signs?

Truck fleet
Posted 22 hours ago

This is the morning
three days after chemo
when the fleet of trucks parks on me…
so, I eat breakfast
take medications
and, go back to bed.

Everything hurts.

I grab my palm cross in my hand
and pray the Lord's Prayer.
Once is not enough.
I am still awake
so I start in again
and probably made it as far as "on earth….as it is in heaven…."
I wake up to my alarm
one hour later.

I go though a "systems check."
How does it feel to move this and this?
How does if feel to breathe?
Everything has improved.

Only one truck remains,
it must have suffered some sort of break down,
because it is parking next to my left shoulder blade
and won't budge.

It's Sunday.
I go back to the Gospel of the day….
I am missing worship
and I am unwilling to miss what God has to say about
these trucks.

The parable of the seeds and the weeds growing amidst them.
I look outside at our own "farm land"
and lots of seed
and plenty of weeds.

And remember last night's rain
and wind
and tiny bits of hail.

Now there is sun,
and rich moist earth.
Those seeds that we planted in the "right places"
are thriving.

But what about those nights with the
hail
and wind
or the mornings with the squirrels digging around them
and the bunnies nibbling at them
and the weeds that I can't keep up with?

If you look at my yard and the garden
you would think the weeds win,
and I am OK with that!

However, when I look at myself,
I am not content with the weed "winning"
I take chemotherapy.
I take medications to make the effects of that chemo disappear
for 4-6 hours at a time.

That truck (and the fleet that parked on me earlier)
is loud
and rude.
But I know something that my medicine doesn't know.

And I know something the truck doesn't know.
And I know something the weeds don't know.
And I know something the cancer doesn't know.

I know another Voice.
I know the Son.
I know that holding that cross each night or each nap
reminds me that I am already being held closely,
regardless of what is growing around me or within me.
Our prayerful conversations remind me
there are no weeds in heaven…
….and we pray "on earth, as it is in heaven."

I go on with my day
knowing the Gardener
will hear my laments about the trucks and weeds
as well as my thanksgivings for medicine and naps and prayer and the
Cross.

That's what I hear this morning.

EPILOGUE

An epilogue. It feels a bit like writing an apology for stopping somewhere in the middle of my story. I guess that is what I want to assure you...and me. That this is the middle. Not the end. The calendar says that it is already five weeks from when I wrote of weeds and trucks. I am still in the same window though. Scans are still two weeks away. Those sometimes offer a plot twist, and sometimes they don't.

But this is all of us, right? We are all in the middle of something, when something else happens. That is where sarcoma found me. Yet, I showed that sarcoma something. I found that God was there -- is here -- Emmanuel, God with us, right in the middle of everything.

In the beginning of writing, I told myself that I wanted people to have the real, correct and true story of what was going on with me. To know what the lab tests said and how I recovered from this procedure and that one. I also wanted to say how I completely rid myself of sarcoma. Some things just don't go as planned.

Nonetheless, I explained things as I learned them. What was hard. What helped. What was beautiful. What I saw from my recliner. What it meant to learn (again and again) to ask for help. What was growing in my garden. What beautiful things I learned to create, in the "face" of something (sarcoma) I never wanted to have created in myself at all.

There are also things that I said little to nothing about, like what it was like to parent young adult children during the perils of the potential loss of another parent. I'm glad to get that thought out there though. If you want to find out how to do that, pray and seek another to help you. That story is one between my dear daughters, and God, and me.

One other thing that is apparent to me today, as the sun shines after a rain is this: I must remember to enjoy and celebrate this glorious middle, this every day-ness, this beauty right here, even in the face of pain. There can be a consuming desire to avoid the end of one's life or peer into it's depths so as to figure it out and control it. Every time I get lost in that fear, I miss the opportunity to give or receive love, to offer or receive care.

Something else quite beautiful is missing from these pages -- it is the collection of responses that people whom I call my "mat carriers" offered to me. My thought is that my writing was my gift to them, and on to you. Their writing was their gift to me. Those who read this on-line were able to see the whole weaving of beautiful mat -- strong and gentle threads, woven together, offering support and love. Yet, this "half-collection" here offers no less, as the your responses, questions, prayers, and notes in the margins become a no-less-treasured gift in a old story made new again.

Breathe. Smile. Pray. Drink your water. Be here now.

"Be strong and of good courage, be neither afraid or dismayed; for the Lord your God is with you wherever you go." Joshua 1:9

ACKNOWLEDGEMENTS

What's with the crying?!

Posted Aug 26, 2014 9:29 a.m.

I have waited so long to write my "Acknowledgements" page. I don't know why I have procrastinated on writing this. I thought maybe it was because I was recovering from chemo....and very sleepy with the meds. But now I know why I wait; it makes me cry -- the whole time! Oh bother!

Try this: (1) Write a list of people or groups of people who have helped you or cared for you in the past three years. (2) Wait 24 hours. Stare at the list every hour or two. (3) The next morning, sit down with your coffee and this list and try to put into words why/how you are thankful for these people/groups of people. (4) If you can do so without weeping, more power to you. I can't. There are a zillion people in the world who would like to have even 5% of the love and support that I have. I am overwhelmed. (5) While you are working on the list and getting the wording just right, talk to God about these people. I compliment God on God's fine work with them. (6) At some point, move the tissue box closer to yourself because it is just going to be annoying to keep reaching so far across the table for it. (7) Tell yourself, "If you just go ahead and type this up you will be one step closer to being done! It is ok if all the words aren't just right. You can proof-read it again!" (8) Bottom line…get over the worry that you will leave out someone's name…or even a whole group of people. That has the capacity to paralyze me and keep me from doing any of this! (9) Pray to remember all their names. (10) Blow your nose. Wipe your tears. (It is yucky if it gets on the computer.) It is worth the tears to let people know they are appreciated.

With thanks to...God -- For your presence. Though I may feel lonely from time to time, I am never alone. For the gift of incredible people in my life -- they are your hands and feet in the world.

Thanks to…Erica -- Though this isn't what you had planned to do after you graduated from college, your creativity in cooking for me, your care of the yard and garden, and the everyday things you do for me are all wonderful gifts.

Sarah -- This has completely changed what your college experience has been like. The added stress has made studying even more difficult, yet you have found your way, selected a rewarding major, and excelled in leadership. Rearranging your schedule with your teachers, and traveling home so often to be with me for chemo and scans are precious gifts.

Rod -- Even though your address is "heaven," your faith, courage, love, and humor are still gifts to us all.

Mom and Dad -- I learned about my faith from you, starting when I was a child, and now no less so as an adult, through your loving care, worship, and prayerfulness. If "heaven and earth" move for me, I know that you have had something to do with it.

Grandma & Grandpa Harding and Grandma & Grandpa Davis -- You personified "grace" for me. I know you are never far away, for God can see us all.

Eric-- You are my treasured brother, child of God, and doctor too, and I am honored to receive your skills in all three areas.

Dorothy Elaine -- For being more than a mother-in-law, for being a living example of hospitality and courage. While you are missed, you are close at heart.

Katherine, Steve, Sue, Bruce, Diana, Dee, Rick -- For helping me continue to have fun, and for helping me stay connected to your wonderful families. It is such a blessing to grow from having one brother -- to having four sisters and four brothers. I'll keep you all.

All my Aunts, Uncles, Cousins, Nieces and Nephews -- Whether you are a few months old, or in you are closer to 90, you are loved. You help me enjoy the things that are a part of every day life -- cookouts, White Elephant gifts, potlucks, springerle cookies, PlayDoh, swimming in the lake, bowling, keeping up on Facebook, a Cubs game at Wrigley Field, walking on South Beach, shopping at Dot's Pots, quilting, hugs and kisses.

Dr. Mo (Mohammed Milhem, MD) -- For being really truly smart...and using that good brain to make a difference for me and so many other people who have sarcoma. You are a wonderful mix of wisdom and caring, and I am thankful for both.

The University of Iowa Holden Cancer Center Staff -- including everyone I encounter from when I register in the cancer center, to lab nurses, the med. techs., the P.A.s, nurse researchers, Wendee the coordinator, Fellows, medical students, pharmacists, infusion center aids and nurses -- ALL of you do what you do so well. It makes a difference for me, and for my family and friends too.

Chaplain Cindy Breed, Dr. Buckwalter, Dr. Iannettoni, Pulmonary Clinic Physicians, CT staff, MRI staff, Cardiac Clinic staff, radiologists and pathologists at the University of Iowa -- You care for so very many people, but when I am in the room, you care for me and my family. Thank you.

The Sarcoma community -- Though this is a community we wish didn't exist, I am thankful for those who have experienced sarcoma before me and participated in clinical trials, and help physicians learn about this cluster of diseases. Thanks as well for offering encouragement and prayers on Facebook. Truly we are connected around the world.

My Clinic Day, Chemo Day, Surgery, & Pulmonary Clinic Day travelers -- In addition to my parents and daughters, I am blessed to have Penny Logan, Dee Brines, Eric & Katherine Harding, Lori Harper, Kellie Duzan, Pat Esker, Stacie Fidlar, Trina Johnston, and Tanya Wittwer travel with me to Iowa City -- It takes a certain bravery and love to come along on these days -- to face whatever might come up and guard your own response so that you can hold me up.

Countless friends, near and far -- The Clinic/Chemo travelers are the tip of the iceberg in terms of the many people praying for and caring for me. These people help me see the best parts of myself and accept the parts that aren't.

Trinity Lutheran Church, Moline, Illinois -- For being a wonderful first-call congregation with a talented staff. For reaching out to me with incredible love and support through this whole trying time, and for gifting me with some of the things I encouraged you to try, including a prayer vigil.

St. John's Lutheran, St. James Lutheran, First Lutheran -- (Rock Island) -- For your welcome and willingness to learn together, with me as your teacher. And, for your leadership in celebrating my ten years of ordained ministry

Mat carriers -- You CarePage readers (who may be listed in another category, too) (individuals and congregations) for holding on to the mat and taking me to Jesus, for offering prayers in your churches and with your friends for almost three years now.

FUNdraiser leaders and participants -- You put your love into action. The funds you raised are still helping me to this day. The joy you created and shared will last a lifetime.

Illinois Wesleyan University in Bloomington, Illinois, Oregon Health Sciences University in Portland, Oregon, Wartburg Seminary in Dubuque, Iowa and St. Paul's Lutheran Church in Warren, Illinois -- For forming me first as a nurse, then as a nursing educator, and then as a pastor. I have needed it all.

Northern Illinois Synod staff -- for your continued prayers, for visits, and for asking how you can help me and colleagues in the future who must travel the murky waters of disability.

Dave Geenan, Stacie Fidlar, Mary Brodd, and St. John's Lutheran Church (RI) -- For your support and expertise in the not-for-profit world, for hosting Living in Hope Foundation as it gets its feet on the ground, and prepares its presence on the web. For understanding the importance of raising money for sarcoma research at University of Iowa.

Editors -- Lyle Ernst & Ann Boaden; Sunflower photographer -- Sheryl Svoboda; Cover designer - Ken Small; and Printing coordinator -- Lori Perkins. For your encouragement, your gracious welcome into this "new world" and your expertise.

For you all, I am not only grateful, I am prayerful: *I thank my God every time I remember you. In all my prayers for all of you, I always pray with joy.* Phil. 1:3-4

References and Suggested Reading or Viewing

Anderson, B., Metzger, B., & Murphy, R. (1991). The new Oxford annotated Bible with the Apocryphal/Deuterocanonical books (1st ed.). New York: Oxford University Press.

Biblical texts used are all New Revised Standard Version (NRSV).

Bard Access Systems, I. (2014). PowerPort* Implantable Port | Implantable Port Devices | Bard Access Systems. Bardaccess.com. Retrieved 19 August 2014, from **http://www.bardaccess.com/port-powerport.php**

While technology is changing all the time, here is the site for the Power Port I have implanted.

Bartlett, D., & Taylor, B. (2008). Feasting on the Word (1st ed.). Louisville: Westminster John Knox Press.

This series of books is written to go along with the three-year Revised Common Lectionary (RCL); it is a favorite preaching resource, and became a devotional tool for me as well.

Bolz-Weber, N. (2013). Pastrix (1st ed.). New York: Jericho Books.

Rev. Nadia Bolz-Weber is an ELCA pastor. The release of her book during my cancer journey gave me another "conversation partner" for some of the big "God questions."

Cameron, J. (2007). Writing diet (1st ed.). New York: Jeremy P. Tarcher/Penguin.

While I did not read this book, it was recommended by Rev. Janet Hunt. I used the "write three long hand pages a day" in addition to writing my CarePage, and yes, I did lose weight!

Clinicaltrials.gov,. (2014). Home - ClinicalTrials.gov. Retrieved 19 August 2014, from **http://www.clinicaltrials.gov**

This is the U.S. Government listing of all clinical trials that are going on. I found my Trabectedin clinical trial listed here.

Evangelical Lutheran Worship. (2006) (1st ed.). Minneapolis: Augsburg Fortress.

I did not list the hymns that I play regularly in the book, but this is the resource I used. I would also read the Psalms or speak some of the liturgy devotionally. The blessing I used on the head of a confirmand is found here in the Affirmation of Faith liturgy.

Evans, R. (2012). The road to grace (1st ed.). New York: Simon & Schuster.

I led a study of this book during the last 3 years. As always, it led to wonderful questions and great conversation. I suggest starting with the first book in this series.

Givetoiowa.org,. (2014). Give Online Now - The University of Iowa Foundation. Retrieved 19 August 2014, from **https://www.givetoiowa.org/GiveToIowa/WebObjects/GiveToIow a.woa/wa/goTo?area=cancer**

This is the site to give directly to Sarcoma Research at the University of Iowa. Proceeds from this book are going here to support Sarcoma Research

Hope, L. (2013). Help me live, revised (1st ed.). Berkeley, Calif...: Celestial Arts.

One of my best friends found this book helpful, especially when I was newly diagnosed. It suggests what to do and what to say.

Hopeonline.tv,. (2014). HOPEONLINE.TV | The Online Campus for Lutheran Church of Hope. Retrieved 19 August 2014, from **http://hopeonline.tv**

Click on "Why Does My Friend Have Cancer?" under the "Since You Asked" sermon series. This is a sermon by the father of another woman who has cancer, Deanna Thompson. She has stage four breast cancer. I reference her book *"Hoping for More."* Her dad is a teaching pastor at Lutheran Church of Hope in West DesMoines Iowa.

Hunt, J. (2013). Dancing with the Word. Dancingwiththeword.com. Retrieved 19 August 2014, from **http://dancingwiththeword.com**

Rev. Janet Hunt writes this commentary (using the RCL) on the scripture(s) for the upcoming week of preaching. Her insights are wonderful, and she engages the reader through thought provoking questions.

Koppenhoefer, L. (2012). Frog Collection. Retrieved from **https://www.youtube.com/watch?v=MnwNSkHArlY**

I reference my Fully Rely On God -- FROG story -- in the book, and made this video of my collection. It is fun for people of all ages.

Koppenhoefer, L. (2011). Membership. Carepages.com. Retrieved 19 August 2014, **www.carepages.com/carepages/LauraKoppyNotesontheJourney**

I started this CarePage soon after I was told I had a tumor in my hip that was most likely cancer. I have written and prayed and grown through the years as I learned to live with sarcoma cancer and with hope. I also experienced a growing concern of the lack of research for this disease.

Koppenhoefer, L. (2013). Mittens of Love. Retrieved from **www.youtube.com/watch?v=5teTQ_YR3xw&feature=youtube**

I was so thrilled to complete my daughter's grey wool cabled fingerless mittens! It was much more complicated than my early washcloth series!

Koppenhoefer, L. (2013). Receiving Grace. Retrieved from **https://www.youtube.com/watch?v=aKYYwJQxjrU**

This is the video that was prepared for a sermon series at St. John's Lutheran Church in Bloomington, Illinois. Rod and I were married at this church and we left it when I went to seminary in 1999.

L'Engle, M., & Chase, C. (1996). Glimpses of grace (1st ed.). [San Francisco]: HarperSanFrancisco.

This collection is a favorite devotional book.

Lewis, C., & Klein, P. (2003). A year with C.S. Lewis (1st ed.). [San Francisco], Calif.: HarperSanFrancisco.

This collection is also a favorite devotional book.

Liddy Shriver Sarcoma Initiative,. (2003). Sarcoma Help | Together we are making a difference!. Retrieved 19 August 2014, from **http://sarcomahelp.org**

This web site was set up by Liddy Shriver's family in Liddy's memory in 2003. Liddy died of sarcoma. The site is one of the "go-to" sites for people who are newly diagnosed -- listing information about the types of sarcoma, sarcoma centers in the U.S.A., information for caregivers and more. They also support sarcoma research.

Lose, D. (2011). Making sense of the cross (1st ed.). Minneapolis: Augsburg Fortress.

This book was used for one of the classes I taught during the break I had from chemotherapy. It is an in depth study of atonement theories -- Biblically, theologically, and experientially. It is written in an engaging dialog format.

Love, J. (2011). Disrupted (1st ed.). Eugene, Or.: Cascade Books.

Julie Anderson Love is a Presbyterian pastor who learns she has an aggressive malignant brain tumor. Her writing pulls you into her challenging physical experience, as well as her wrestling with God.

Luther, M., & Owen, B. (1998). Jesus, remember me (1st ed.). Minneapolis: Augsburg.

This small book is a simple comfort in days when long words and complicated prayers won't do -- like when your loved one has died....or you are diagnosed with cancer.

Mayo Clinic,. (2014). Soft tissue sarcoma Symptoms - Diseases and Conditions - Mayo Clinic. Mayoclinic.com. Retrieved 19 August 2014 **http://www.mayoclinic.com/health/soft-tissue-sarcoma/DS00601/DSECTION=symptoms**

This Mayo Clinic resource is very helpful for understanding sarcoma and its many symptoms.

Milhem, M. (2013). Melanoma and Sarcoma | Mo. Doctormoiowa.wordpress.com. Retrieved 19 August 2014, from **http://doctormoiowa.wordpress.com/category/melanoma-and-sarcoma/**

Dr. Mohammed Milhem -- Dr. Mo, for short -- is my sarcoma specialist oncologist. He is likely one of the most brilliant people I have ever met. His blog reveals his deep caring for people, and the stresses that are inherent to his role. Many people guest-write and offer interesting perspectives.

Nouwen, H. (1997). Bread for the journey (1st ed.). San Francisco: Harper SanFrancisco.

This is another favorite devotional book.

Remen, R. (2006). Kitchen table wisdom (1st ed.). New York: Riverhead Books.

This is an insightful book by Dr. Remen -- with perspectives from her medical practice, and her own experience with chronic disease.

Schwiebert, P., DeKlyen, C., & Bills, T. (1999). Tear soup (1st ed.). Portland, Or.: Grief Watch.

This beautifully illustrated book is for children of all ages -- with hopes of comforting those who grieve.

Thompson, D. (2012). Hoping for more (1st ed.). Eugene, Or: Cascade Books.

This professor of religion writes about her experience with stage IV breast cancer -- as a wife, mother, professor, friend. She thinks deeply about her disease and relationship with God.

Thompson, D. (2014). hoping for more. Hopingformore.com. Retrieved 19 August 2014, from **http://hopingformore.com**

This web site links information about Deanna Thompson and her book by the same name as her site.

Wangerin, W. (2010). Letters from the land of cancer (1st ed.). Grand Rapids, Mich.: Zondervan.

Walter Wangerin, Jr. Writes of his experience of lung cancer in letters to family and friends.

Whitcomb, H. (2005). Seven spiritual gifts of waiting (1st ed.). Minneapolis: Augsburg Books.

I have taught this book for four congregations -- and it was worth it every time. There is so much waiting in everyone's life -- in mine as I taught, I was waiting for test results, or for treatments to work, or for a daughter to come home from college. The reader explores where God and one's faith are in the waiting as well.